WHY DO I FEEL LIKE S#!T?

The 5 stupidly simple steps to balance your mood and hormones.

N'Jaane Taylor

Supported by Dr. Ces Franks

About Your Author

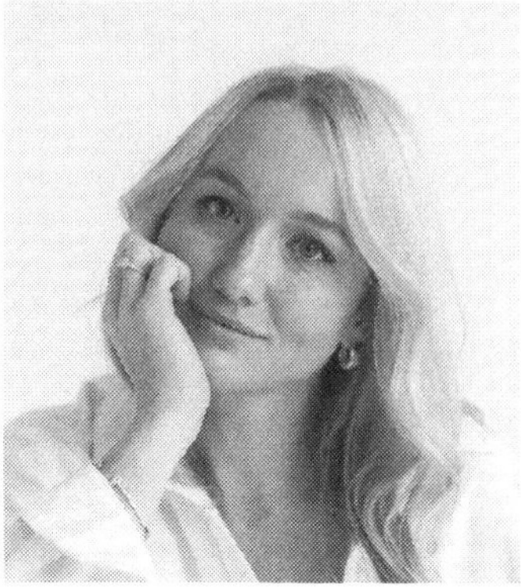

N'Jaane Taylor doesn't offer clichés or quick fixes. She's an Integrative Nutrition practitioner with a unique approach rooted in addressing the core issues that hold you back: a dysregulated nervous system, unresolved trauma, and the subconscious patterns steering your life. This insight has become the cornerstone of her work, weaving together nutrition, neuroscience and breathwork to help women reconnect with their bodies.

At just 17, N'Jaane faced homelessness—a moment that could have shattered her. Instead, it shaped her. From professional dancer to nationally touring DJ, she built a life that defied the odds, even as she silently battled the chronic pain of adenomyosis and endometriosis. These challenges didn't just test her—they taught her. The tools she created to survive and thrive formed the backbone of her groundbreaking work.

When her mother was diagnosed with stage 3 endometrial cancer, N'Jaane left her performance career to step fully into her calling: helping women rebuild their relationship with their bodies. This mission led to the creation of Unprocessed, an app blending nutrition and neuroscience to balance hormones, mood and chronic dysregulation within the body. Unprocessed isn't just an app—it's a movement, with profits set to fund research in women's reproductive health, groundbreaking work in oncological nutrition and utilising the data to drive these studies and discover meaningful solutions that further assist her Unprocessed community.

About Your Author

As the author of Why Do I Feel Like Shit?, N'Jaane combines science, wit, and raw honesty into a no-nonsense guide to understanding your nervous system, rewriting subconscious patterns, and reclaiming your life. Her work isn't about perfection; it's about progress, balance, and finding a way forward that feels true to you.

N'Jaane isn't here to fix you—because you're not broken. She's here to walk alongside you, offering tools, compassion, and a steady hand as you navigate the often messy, always rewarding process of healing. You don't have to do it alone.

njt

Pinterest: @njaanetaylor
Instagram: @njaanetaylor
TikTok: @njaanetaylor
YouTube: @njaanetaylor

Edition #1
First Published by N'Jaane Taylor in 2024

ISBN 978-1-7637609-0-5

Cover design by N'Jaane Taylor
Typeset in 10 / 16 Corbel
Printed and bound in Australia by Mixam Printing

This book is dedicated to, **you**.
Your commitment to creating a safe space for yourself.
You're amazing, and I am proud of you.

And when it gets hard, please don't give up.
I am in your corner.

Disclaimer:

This book has been written to offer general advice and broad information on nutrition, lifestyle and neuroscience topics and is not a replacement for professional help. While implementing the strategies outlined in this book can be helpful, it does not replace speaking to a professional or seeking help from your doctor. If you feel that you are suffering from a mental or physical disorder, or if you have experienced any kind of trauma, this book is designed and intended to be a supportive aid, please seek further help and guidance to support yourself safely in your healing journey.

P.s:

This book has been formatted whilst watching the final season of Yellowstone, apologies in advance for any mistakes... sorry not sorry.

Index:

Read the whole thing - trust the process.

Establishing Your Safe Space: A Portable Resource.

Establishing Your Safe Space: A Portable Resource

Hi, I'm N'Jaane Taylor, and I'm a recovering people-pleaser with a PhD in overthinking. In writing these pages, I unearthed knowledge and personal insights that have shaped my own healing journey, it's my heartfelt hope that they will offer the same support to you. Together, we'll navigate the next 220-ish pages with curiosity, courage, and a touch of humour.

This book is designed to be your anchor—a steady presence during the storms of healing, whether you're embarking on this path alone or with the guidance of a practitioner. These pages are here to guide you back to safety, to homeostasis, and / or to a state of 'okay-ness' when difficult triggers arise. In time, and with the tools shared here, you'll become your own unwavering resource—a safe harbour within yourself. You'll learn to trust that no matter what emotions come your way, you can weather them. Your nervous system will grow as serene and steady as a dawn-lit lake on a crisp autumn morning... most of the time.
Until then, let this book be your companion.

It's ok to feel anxious. It's ok to feel sad. It's even ok to have dark thoughts. These emotions are not the enemy. When we stop resisting them and allow ourselves to truly feel, we open the door to healing. By letting the waves of emotion crash over us, anchored and steady, we realise we can endure the storm. Just as every storm passes, so too will these emotions. You are strong enough to feel an emotion without becoming it. Sometimes, the most profound act of healing is sitting with discomfort and allowing it to move through your body, rather than over-intellectualising the process.

Establishing Your Safe Space: A Portable Resource

Your body, with its remarkable intelligence, breathes, moves, and heals without any conscious effort or acknowledgment. It's only when uncomfortable emotions such as anxiety, sadness or anger surface that we begin to take notice.
Next time these emotions arise, shift your attention from your thoughts to your body. How does the feeling manifest physically?
Sit with it. Learn about it. Maybe even befriend it.
Emotions are the wormholes to healing, and the only way out is through.

If facing these emotions feels overwhelming, that's ok too.
Healing doesn't demand perfection or haste.
Sometimes, we need to focus on coping—finding tools that bring immediate relief—before we're ready to fully heal. Whether it's practicing with a professional or easing in with less intense emotions, take the time you need to build trust within yourself.

When it all feels overwhelming, this book—and the portable resource we're about to create together—can serve as your safety blanket, offering comfort and steadiness when you need it most.

Establishing Your Safe Space: A Portable Resource

Your Written or Visual Safety Blanket—a tool for dealing.

Think of a memory or place that instantly brings you a sense of calm and safety—a moment where you felt grounded, at ease, and fully secure within yourself. It could be a peaceful nature spot, a childhood home or even a favorite activity where you feel most connected to yourself.
It can also be a place that you curate in your own mind.

You can choose to write about it in detail or find a photo (or several) that represents this safe space. Use the space provided on the next two pages for your words or images. This is your personal sanctuary, a resource you can turn to whenever life feels overwhelming.

When feelings of anxiety, stress, or disconnection arise, and it is too overwhelming to feel, open these pages and bring yourself back to this place. Let this visual or written anchor remind you of the inner strength and security that already resides within you. It's a grounding touchstone to help bring you back to your centre.

Feeling Numb or Dissociated?
If you begin to feel numb or dissociated, try gently shaking your body, stretching, or even dancing in a private space. Movement can help you reconnect with your body and the present moment, guiding you back to a place of balance.

Remember, this is your journey. Your safe space lives within you.

Nervous System.

Nervous System

By now, the term "nervous system" has likely graced your ears as frequently as your favourite tune. Whether from the mouths of friends, healthcare professionals, or that oh-so-persuasive biohacker who insists that intermittent fasting will unlock your brain's full potential, the nervous system is undeniably having a moment. This newfound attention is well-deserved, as this complex network is not just a backdrop to your existence but rather the conductor of the symphony that is your body. It can, depending on how well it's regulated, either compose a harmonious masterpiece or plunge you into discordant chaos.

However, before we continue to heap praise on this biological maestro, let's assess your understanding. Are you, perhaps, already fluent in the language of neurons and synapses? If so, congratulations, dear scholar—feel free to advance to the next chapter, where I will personally commend your alacrity with a virtual handshake. But if your familiarity with the nervous system is more akin to a vague acquaintance, then stay with me; we have much to explore.

Nervous System 101: Your Body's Own Telegram Network

There's no need to be intimidated by the nervous system. Imagine it as an intricate telegraph system from the days of yore, where messages zipped between distant outposts with remarkable speed and efficiency. In a modern twist, your brain is the central hub, dispatching messages through a vast network of nerves and cells to the farthest reaches of your body, including those enigmatic organs. Think of it like your local café: you might not converse with every patron, but Tom is always eager to entertain you with tales of Cheryl's weekend adventures, ensuring that, in this cosy microcosm, everyone remains connected. Similarly, your nervous system's nerves act as messengers, linking your brain and spinal cord to various parts of your body, coordinating every action from the mundane to the miraculous.

The Brain: The Sovereign of the Central Nervous System
At the heart of the Central Nervous System (CNS) lies the brain, the sovereign ruler of your bodily realm. This organ, a masterpiece of biological engineering, presides over all that you see, think, and feel. It is divided into distinct regions, each as crucial as the next: the cerebrum, which governs thought and memory; the cerebellum, the guardian of balance and coordination; and the brainstem, the tireless overseer of vital functions like breathing and heart rate. The brain is your personal control centre, where all decisions—be they monumental or trivial—are made with impeccable precision.

The spinal cord is the brain's trusted emissary, a superhighway of neural pathways that connects the brain to every organ and body part. Picture it as the grand boulevard of your nervous system, where messages are relayed with unerring accuracy and speed, ensuring that the body functions as a cohesive whole.

The Peripheral Nervous System (PNS) is akin to the king's messengers, delivering the brain's edicts to the farthest corners of the kingdom a.k.a. your body. This sprawling network branches out from the CNS, reaching every limb and organ to ensure that no cell is left unconnected.
This PNS is composed of two main divisions:

1. **The Somatic Nervous System (SNS):** The SNS is responsible for voluntary movements—everything you consciously decide to do, from strolling through a park, raising a glass of wine or typing a witty response to a text. The SNS transmits orders from the brain to your skeletal muscles, directing them to contract or relax in

response to your will. Whether you're playing a sonata on the piano, picking up a cup of coffee, or dramatically tossing your hair over your shoulder, the SNS is at work, executing your every command with military precision.

2. **The Autonomic Nervous System (ANS):** The ANS is the unsung hero of your body's operations, overseeing all those vital functions that occur without your conscious input. Heart rate, digestion, respiratory rhythm—these are all the ANS's domain. It's like the loyal butler who keeps the estate running smoothly, handling everything from the temperature of the drawing-room to the timing of the meals, all without bothering you for a single instruction.

Autonomic Nervous System: The Three Pillars of Autonomy
Within the ANS, there exist three distinct systems, each with its own role in maintaining your body's internal harmony:

A) **Sympathetic Nervous System:** The sympathetic system is the body's alarm bell, ever ready to spring into action at the first sign of danger. When faced with stress, fear, or a situation requiring immediate response, this system floods your body with norepinephrine and epinephrine, increasing your heart rate, dilating your pupils, and directing blood to your muscles—all the better to fight or flee.

B) **Parasympathetic Nervous System:** The parasympathetic system is the body's calming influence, the counterpart to the sympathetic system's intensity. It's responsible for bringing your body back to a state of rest and digestion after a stressful event. The vagus nerve, the crowning jewel of this system, plays a crucial role in regulating heart rate, digestion, and social engagement. It's like the gentle touch of a skilled therapist, coaxing your body into relaxation and restoring balance after a stormy episode. It is important to note that this 'chill' sector of the nervous system can also be responsible for the 'shutdown' or 'freeze' response. We will take a deep dive into the specifics of this shortly.

C) **Enteric Nervous System:** Often referred to as the "second brain," the enteric nervous system governs your gastrointestinal tract with a remarkable degree of autonomy. Though it operates independently, it remains under the influence of both the sympathetic and parasympathetic systems. It's the chef in your body's kitchen, ensuring that every meal is digested efficiently and that nutrients are absorbed with precision.

Nervous System

Key Components: The Nobility of the Nervous System

Let's delve into the specific players in this grand performance:

- **Cranial Nerves:** Like a council of advisors, these 12 pairs of nerves emerge directly from the brain, each with its own sphere of influence, from the optic nerves that grant you sight to the facial nerves that enable expression.
- **Spinal Nerves:** With 31 pairs in total, spinal nerves branch out from the spinal cord, serving specific regions of your body. They're like the local delivery service, ensuring every part of your body gets its brain messages on time.
- **Sensory and Motor Nerves:** Sensory nerves carry information from your skin, muscles, and organs back to the CNS, while motor nerves take the CNS's orders to your muscles and glands. It's a bit like sending a postcard to your brain and getting a reply via express mail.
- **Autonomic Nerves:** These include the sympathetic and parasympathetic fibres that innervate organs and control those all-important involuntary functions. They're like the behind-the-scenes crew in a theatre production—working tirelessly to keep the show running smoothly.

The Peripheral Nervous System, with its somatic and autonomic divisions, is the communication network that links the Central Nervous System to every part of your body. It is the sophisticated infrastructure that enables you to think, move, feel, and survive. Next time someone mentions their nervous system, you can nod knowingly, secure in the knowledge that you're not only familiar with this intricate system—you're practically on a first-name basis with it.

Nervous System

What Happens in Vagus, Does Not Stay in Vagus.

Ah, the vagus nerve, a rather distinguished member of our cranial entourage. As the tenth cranial nerve, the vagus (Latin for "wandering") nerve is, quite aptly, the longest of the cranial nerves. It meanders with the grace of a well-travelled aristocrat, extending its influence over a substantial portion of the parasympathetic nervous system—a solid approximately 75%, no less. Now, within this marvel of biological design, we find a trio of distinct yet interrelated parts:

1. **Dorsal Vagus (Low Tone):** Rest and Digest
   This branch is the quintessential bearer of calm, soothing signals. When this low-tone dorsal vagus takes charge, the body is gently lulled into a state of rest and digestion, like a peaceful countryside retreat where everything slows to a leisurely pace. This is the parasympathetic system at its most tranquil, ensuring that our meals are digested with the utmost care, and our energy is conserved for more pressing matters.

2. **Dorsal Vagus (High Tone):** Freeze and Immobilisation
   A change in tone, however, and the story takes a darker turn. The high-tone dorsal vagus is the harbinger of the freeze response, a survival mechanism as ancient as life itself. When faced with an overwhelming threat, the body, under this high-tone influence, may become immobilised—a strategy born of last resort, akin to playing dead in the hopes of evading a predator's gaze.

3. **Ventral Vagus:** Connect and Engage
   Finally, we come to the ventral vagus, a nerve that might be considered the socialite of the bunch. This branch is all about connection, engagement, and the warm fuzzies of human interaction. It's the ventral vagus that enables us to smile at a friend,

feel at ease in conversation, or connect deeply with another person. It's the nerve that fosters the social bonds that are so vital to our well-being.

Let's not forget the nerve's more practical duties: The vagus nerve is a master communicator, relaying signals between the brain, heart, and digestive system. Should this nerve suffer damage—oh, the horror!—one might experience gastroparesis, where food stubbornly refuses to vacate the stomach and move along into the intestines, causing a rather unpleasant state of affairs.

Now, while the vagus nerve operates within the autonomous realm of the autonomic nervous system—where it usually does its work without requiring our conscious input—it is not entirely beyond our influence. Through various practices, such as deep breathing, meditation, and even certain dietary choices, we can gently coax the vagus nerve into favouring its more benevolent roles. Thus, we can ensure that this wandering nerve continues its vital work, promoting a state of harmony within our complex internal symphony.

Nervous System

Your Nervous Systems Daily Rituals:

1. **Response to Stress**
   Picture this: You're late for a meeting, your coffee's gone cold, and your phone's at 2% battery. Your body's "fight-or-flight" response kicks in, ready to turn you into either a superhero or a track star. Understanding this stress mechanism helps you know when to hit pause so that you don't end up in a permanent state of "I can't even." Recognising when your body needs a break can be the difference between gracefully bowing out and a full-blown meltdown - I will admit to be talking out of experience on this one.

2. **Mental Health**
   Neurotransmitters are your brain's text messages, controlling everything from mood to sleep. When these messages get scrambled, you can end up with anxiety, depression, or insomnia. Understanding this can help you realise when your brain's inbox is full, and it's time to clear out the junk mail with a little self-care or professional help.

3. **Movement and Coordination**
   Ever tried to dance and ended up looking like a wacky inflatable tube man? That's your nervous system trying to coordinate all those fancy moves. It's in charge of every step, twirl, and accidental trip. Getting to know how it works can help you fine-tune your motor skills or at least give you a heads-up when something's off-kilter.

Nervous System

4. **Sensory Perception**
   Your nervous system is the backstage crew for your five senses—sight, hearing, touch, taste, and smell. It's the reason you can enjoy the aroma of freshly brewed coffee or wince at your neighbour's out-of-tune singing. It's like having your very own backstage pass to the world, interpreting everything and giving you a front-row seat to life's sensory experiences.

5. **Learning and Memory**
   The brain's basically your internal Wikipedia, storing and retrieving information at lightning speed. Understanding how it manages this encyclopaedia of knowledge can help you optimise your study habits, ensuring you don't draw a blank when it's time to show off your smarts. Plus, it might just help you remember where you left your keys.

6. **Nutrition and Digestion**
   Your nervous system has a say in everything from when you feel hungry to how well you digest that burger. Knowing how it influences your appetite and digestion can lead to better meal choices—because let's face it, a happy gut makes for a happy life.

7. **Pain Management**
   Pain is your body's way of saying, "Hey, something's not right!" Understanding how your nervous system transmits these signals can help you manage pain more effectively, like finding the best strategy to deal with that stubborn headache. It's not about ignoring the pain but learning how to respond to it in a way that doesn't involve curling up in a ball and hoping it'll go away.

Nervous System

Practical Examples

- **Stress Management**: Knowing how your nervous system reacts to stress can inspire you to embrace meditation, exercise, or even a good nap to keep your inner drama queen in check.
- **Healthy Habits**: Understanding how your nervous system handles hunger can motivate you to stick to regular meal times, making "hangry" a thing of the past.
- **Mental Well-being**: Awareness of your brain's chemistry can lead to better mental health practices, like maintaining social connections or diving into hobbies that light up your world.

Remember, the nervous system is the conductor of your body's orchestra, ensuring every part plays its role in harmony. By understanding how it works, you can make smarter choices for your overall well-being. Whether it's recognizing when to chill out, adopting healthier habits, or seeking help when things go off track, this knowledge empowers you to lead a healthier, happier life. Plus, you'll have some impressive facts to drop at your next dinner party.

Trying to out think your Nervous System.

Trying to out think your Nervous System

Ah, the noble pursuit of reason, forever outmatched by the tempestuous tides of emotion. Picture, if you will, the delicate dance between the brain's limbic system—the very cradle of our emotional existence—and the prefrontal cortex, that bastion of logic and reason. Alas, when the limbic system seizes the reins, your rational thoughts become mere spectators in the wild theatre of emotional upheaval.

In moments of nervous system dysregulation, when one is thrust into the throes of fight, flight, freeze, or fawn, the body becomes a veritable fortress in survival mode. Here, the limbic system (we're talking emotions darling) commands the stage, while the logic and demure of the prefrontal cortex is relegated to the back row, clutching its pearls. Imagine, if you will, attempting to negotiate with a fire alarm. You may wax poetic about the absence of flames, but the alarm, in its fervent duty, cares not for reason. It will continue to wail, for it perceives a threat, real or imagined. Similarly, when your nervous system is thrown into disarray, emotional reactions are already in motion before your rational brain even has a chance to flex its thinking cap.

Why such haste, you ask?
A lifetime of evolution has fine-tuned this emotional machinery and nervous system to work at the speed of light—or at least as close as biology can muster in order to protect us from danger. By the time you have consciously registered the emotional reaction, your body has already unleashed a battalion of stress hormones like cortisol and adrenaline, prepping you for the perceived threat.

Attempting to out think an emotional response is akin to instructing oneself not to flinch at a sudden noise—charming in theory, but utterly implausible in practice. Rather than wrestling with the inevitable, the

key lies in acknowledging the emotion, soothing your nervous system (through techniques such as deep breathing or grounding exercises), and only then summoning your rational faculties to make sense of it all.
In short, dear reader, you cannot simply logic your way out of a nervous system in crisis mode. Instead, focus first on calming the body, and the mind, like a loyal servant, will follow in due course.
When it comes to calming your body, there are two approaches you can take:

Option A: Healing
This involves letting that uncomfortable emotion exist in your body rather than wrestling with it like an uninvited guest overstaying their welcome. Your body needs to feel these sensations in order to process them. As a practical example, I step out of my mind and into my body by doing a head-to-toe scan, simply noticing whatever sensation pops up. For me, this often feels like my heart is auditioning for a drum solo, while my stomach ties itself into Olympic-level knots. There was a time when this feeling was utterly overwhelming—like my body was a ticking time bomb—and it would send me into a spiral of panic, feeling completely out of control.

With practice, I've sort of...befriended the sensation. Yep, you can actually get comfortable with it. I've learned to sit with the feeling, and spoiler alert: it gets easier. Think of anxiety as just another physical sensation, much like the sharp pain of stubbing your toe. The key difference? We accept toe pain with a groan and a hop, but we wage war against the discomfort of anxiety. Learning to feel safe within this sensation is like unlocking a secret level in a video game—suddenly, calm resilience is available to you, even in the midst of chaos.

Trying to out think your Nervous System

Fair warning: Option A does take time and practice. In the beginning, it's best done with a trauma-informed practitioner such as myself who can guide you through the process. While you're working on that, allow me to introduce you to **Option B.**

Option B: Dealing

This is the art of gracefully directing your mind and body away from the perceived threat and toward a place of safety. This safe space can be anything—an uplifting memory, your favourite song, a photo that makes you smile—anything that brings you back to a grounded, secure feeling. You'll find a handy step-by-step guide in the first few pages of this book on how to create your own personal safe space, ready to anchor you whenever a storm starts brewing. Trust me, it's like giving your brain its very own "Do Not Disturb" sign.

The essence of growth lies in mastering the space between stimulus and response—it's that magical pause where real transformation happens. In this space, we are allowing our emotions to come, being present and feeling what we need to feel without acting through it; we're waiting until the emotional and animalistic response of the limbic system passes, enabling the elegant and calm prefrontal cortex to assume charge and consciously choose our response, allowing for a moment of clarity and purpose.

Trying to out think your Nervous System

I particularly love the principle of **PAUSE**:

- **P**ause: Take a moment to step back. Before you react, allow yourself a brief intermission.
- **A**ction: Don't jump into action right away. Let the impulse simmer down.
- **U**ntil: Wait until you've regained a sense of calm.
- **S**erenity: Only then should you move forward, guided by a sense of peace.
- **E**nters: Let this serenity guide your next steps, ensuring your actions are measured and thoughtful.

This method encourages us to embrace our emotions fully, but without being enslaved by them. Instead of letting emotions drive our decisions, we allow space for calm and clarity to lead the way. This approach not only fosters personal growth but also leads to more mindful and effective responses to life's challenges.

Flicking the Nervous System Switch.

Flicking the Nervous System Switch

Alright, darling, let's set the stage: Picture yourself, comfy in your favourite oversized sweater, snuggled up with a bucket of popcorn, eyes glued to a horror movie. Suddenly, without warning, a ghastly figure lunges from the screen. Your heart begins to hammer in your chest as if you're auditioning for a role in an action film. Your breathing turns erratic, and you're mentally preparing yourself to either sprint out of the room or karate-chop the TV. Welcome to the sympathetic nervous system's debut—the star of the show when it comes to "fight or flight."

But then, as the credits roll, the lights flick back on, and you remember it's just a movie (or is it?). The adrenaline-fueled warrior in you gives way to a more serene version, ready to return to reality, sip some tea, and actually chill. Enter the parasympathetic nervous system, the unassuming yet indispensable hero that ushers you back to calm waters—a state I'll dub "Netflix and genuinely chill."

This magical transformation isn't just for show; it's a real biological process known as **autonomic balance** or **autonomic regulation**. Imagine it as your body's way of saying, "Alright, drama Lama, time to settle down and return to the land of the living."
Here's how the show goes on:

1. Heart Rate Cool-Down

- **The Drama:** You receive an unexpected email from your boss, or worse, a surprise text from your ex. Cue the sympathetic nervous system, racing your heart as though you're about to run a marathon. Your body is ready to tackle whatever stress comes its way.

- **The How:** Your brain hits the panic button, signalling your adrenal glands to pump out adrenaline, which nudges your heart into overdrive. Your muscles are suddenly poised for action, just in case you need to channel your inner Wonder Woman.

- **Post-Drama:** Once the coast is clear, the parasympathetic nervous system takes the reins, releasing acetylcholine—a neurotransmitter that coos to your heart, "Chill, babe, you've got this," bringing your heart rate down to a more leisurely pace.

2. Blood Vessel Tranquility

- **The Drama:** When stress strikes, your blood vessels tighten up, redirecting blood to your muscles—think of it as your body's way of preparing for battle, be it with a zombie or a looming deadline.

- **The How:** The sympathetic system enlists noradrenaline to constrict your blood vessels, ensuring that every drop of blood is ready to fuel your fight or flight.

- **Post-Drama:** As the drama subsides, nitric oxide—a delightful molecule of peace—emerges, prompting your blood vessels to relax and open up. The result? Better blood flow, improved digestion, and an overwhelming sense of relief.

3. Smooth Muscle Relaxation

- **The Drama:** In the midst of chaos, digestion takes a backseat. Your body, laser-focused on survival, decides that your sandwich can wait.

- **The How:** Stress hormones like adrenaline and noradrenaline signal your digestive system to pause, contracting smooth muscles and putting your digestion on hold.

- **Post-Drama:** Once the crisis is averted, acetylcholine steps back in to soothe those muscles, resuming normal digestion. Now, you can finally enjoy that sandwich without a care in the world.

4. Stress Hormone Detox

- **The Drama:** Stress hormones like cortisol and adrenaline flood your system, providing that quick burst of energy you need to conquer the task at hand.
- **The How:** The sympathetic system sends a distress call to your adrenal glands, which responds by releasing these potent hormones. Your body is officially on high alert.
- **Post-Drama:** The parasympathetic system helps to cleanse your system of these hormones, allowing you to unwind and preventing the detrimental effects of prolonged stress.

The Brain's Leading Roles in Stress and Relaxation

Hypothalamus: The grandmaster, orchestrating the shift between the high-stakes action of the sympathetic system and the cool-down routine of the parasympathetic system. Imagine it as the ultimate DJ, spinning tracks to match the vibe—whether you're in a club (aka stress mode) or at a spa (aka relaxation).

Amygdala: The danger detector, and mediator of emotion.
A small, almond-shaped structure inside of your brain. Working as the ever-watchful sentinel, scanning for threats, whether real or imaginary (like that email from your boss at 2am). It's the one that yells, "Fight or flight, folks!" the moment it senses danger.

Flicking the Nervous System Switch

Prefrontal Cortex: The brain's wise counsel, tempering the amygdala's hysteria with logic and reason. It's like that friend who calmly reminds you that maybe, just maybe, that horror movie was just a movie.

Hippocampus: The memory keeper, reminding you that you've survived this before, whether it's a horror flick or a stressful situation. It provides context, helping you keep calm and carry on.

In short, this elegant shift from "fight or flight" to "chill mode" is your body's way of maintaining balance, ensuring you don't remain a bundle of nerves indefinitely. So, the next time your heart races at the sight of a shadowy figure or an unexpected email, remember—your body's got your back, and it's ready to guide you back to serenity as soon as the drama fades.

Hormones.

Hormones

In this book, I'll be delving into a variety of hormones—how they're produced, how they're secreted, and the crucial roles they play in keeping your body's inner workings in top-notch condition. But before we get ahead of ourselves, let's tackle the big question: what exactly is a hormone?

A hormone is a chemical that acts as a set of instructions, produced by specific glands in your body—we are talking thyroid, adrenal glands, and pancreas. Imagine this chemical as a detailed memo sent to a cell or organ, informing it to kick-start or halt a particular process. These physiological processes oversee everything from growth, metabolism, and mood to the operation of your organs, essentially playing a pivotal role in the seamless functionality of your body. All clear?

In more relatable terms, consider hormones as your body's version of text messages. Just like you shoot a quick message to your friends to share the latest scoop, your body dispatches these chemical messages through your bloodstream. These messages, crafted by special glands, provide your cells and organs with the latest updates and instructions.

For instance, some hormones might signal your body to sprout a few more inches, ramp up your energy levels, or even influence your mood (ever wondered why you sometimes feel a bit off-kilter? That's hormones at work!). Much like the banter in a group chat with your besties, hormones help your body stay in sync and operate smoothly. So, the next time you feel a surge of energy or a sudden mood swing, remember it's just your body's way of sending crucial "texts" about what it needs—be it a boost, a break, or a bit of downtime. Instead of fighting this mystical world of bodily communication, it is time to learn how to listen to it, support it and work with it rather than against it.

Hormones

How the Nervous System Plays with Your Hormones (that sounded better in my head)

Understanding how your nervous system and hormones team up is like getting the VIP pass to your body's very own reality show—a chaotic mix of dramatic highs, lows, and everything in between. Picture your life as an episode of "Hormones Gone Wild," where your emotions are the unpredictable stars, throwing tantrums and having emotional breakdowns one minute, then making up and being besties the next. This is all thanks to the behind-the-scenes directors: your nervous system and hormones. If you are already somewhat of a hormone expert, this won't be any new information to you, however the analogies are golden and I still recommend reading for giggles.

Neurotransmitters and Hormones: The Dynamic Duo

In our era of instant gratification, think of neurotransmitters as the fast-typing friend who DMs you the gossip the second it happens. Meanwhile, hormones are the more reserved pal who sends a thoughtful group text, making sure everyone's in the loop. It is important to note that they can also multi-task, take norepinephrine for instance—it's the friend who can't decide whether to be that speedy neurotransmitter messenger or the hormone taking the more laid-back group chat route.

Hypothalamus-Pituitary Axis: The Brain's Command Centre

The hypothalamus is the diva of your brain, managing everything from your stress response to how quickly you burn through that last cupcake. It sends orders to the pituitary gland, which then delegates tasks to other glands such as your thyroid and adrenal glands. Think of it as the ultimate multitasker, overseeing your body's day-to-day operations with the efficiency of a highly caffeinated CEO.

Hormones

Stress Response: From Freakout to Chill

When you're faced with a stressful situation—like running late for a big event or accidentally sending a message to the wrong group chat—your nervous system sends an SOS to your adrenal glands. They respond by flooding your system with adrenaline and cortisol, kicking you into "I got this" mode. Your heart races, your senses sharpen, and suddenly you're ready to take on the world—or at least tackle that stressful situation head-on.

Feedback Loops: Keeping Everything in Check

Your nervous system is like that overprotective friend who constantly checks in to make sure everything's under control. It monitors your hormone levels, making sure none of them get too dramatic. If one hormone starts acting out, your nervous system sends a polite but firm message to the relevant gland, telling it to chill out and keep things balanced... when it is regulated.

Growth and Metabolism: The Behind-the-Scenes Heroes

Your thyroid hormones are like the backstage crew of a concert—they're not in the spotlight, but without them, nothing would go smoothly. These hormones ensure your brain develops properly, your metabolism hums along, and you don't turn into a hangry gremlin. They're the unsung heroes that keep your body in tip-top shape.

Reproduction: Hormones and All the Feels

Hormones like oestrogen, progesterone and testosterone aren't just in charge of your reproductive system—they're also the ones messing with your mood, energy levels, and brainpower. When they're in balance, you're feeling great, but when they're not, well... cue the emotional rollercoaster. One minute you're feeling like a queen, and the next, you're questioning all your life choices.

Mood and Cognition: Hormones That Run the Show

Cortisol, oestrogen, progesterone and testosterone are the headliners in your mood and mental clarity. For instance, oestrogen, when balanced, is your personal life coach—when it's regulated, you're feeling upbeat and sharp but when it drops, suddenly everything feels a bit foggy, and your mood might take a nosedive. Understanding these hormones is like getting a peek behind the curtain of your own emotional and mental state.

The Hypothalamus and Pituitary Gland: Name a more iconic Duo

These two are the Beyoncé and Jay-Z of your body's hormonal system. The hypothalamus calls the shots, while the pituitary gland makes sure the orders are carried out by the rest of your glands. Together, they keep everything running smoothly, from your metabolism to your stress response.

The Fight-or-Flight Response: Your Inner Warrior

When life throws a curveball, your nervous system is like a superhero, rallying your adrenal glands to release adrenaline and cortisol. These hormones boost your heart rate, sharpen your senses, and give you the energy to handle whatever comes your way. It's your body's way of saying, "You've got this!"

Nutrition and Your Nervous System: A Three-Part Story

Your hypothalamus is the mastermind behind your hunger cues, sending messages to your brain when you're hungry or full. It's the voice in your head that says, "Maybe don't have that third slice of cake." Meanwhile, the enteric nervous system is your gut's personal assistant, managing everything from digestion to nutrient absorption. When it comes to blood sugar, your nervous system coordinates with your pancreas to keep everything in check, ensuring you have the energy you need without crashing.

Putting It All Together: The Ultimate Power Couple

Think of your body as a luxury car, with the nervous system as the driver and hormones as the finely tuned engine. Together, they keep everything running smoothly, ensuring you have the energy to tackle the day, the focus to stay on top of your game, and the resilience to handle whatever life throws your way.

Cognition and Mood: Explained

Your hormones aren't just about making sure your body runs smoothly—they also have a huge impact on how you feel and think. We will dive deeper into this in one moment.

The Brain-Hormone Tango

Picture this: your hormones and neurotransmitters are at a lively dance party in your brain. Cortisol, oestrogen, progesterone, and testosterone are on the guest list, each with their own dance style, shaking things up in the most intriguing ways.

Hormones

Cortisol is that one guest who turns up when things get stressful. Like a caffeine-fueled party crasher, it gives you a burst of energy to tackle immediate challenges. Beware, if cortisol overstays its welcome, it can leave your brain feeling frazzled, foggy, and forgetful—like the morning after a wild night out.
Cortisol is the go-to hormone for stress management, providing you with a burst of energy when needed. But like that friend who can be a bit too intense, too much cortisol can leave you feeling anxious, irritable, and even a bit down. It can mess with your sleep, zap your energy, and make concentrating feel like a Herculean task.

Oestrogen is the elegant ballroom dancer of the group, gracefully enhancing memory and learning. When oestrogen levels are just right, everything feels in sync, like you're effortlessly gliding across the dance floor. But when oestrogen decides to sit out a few songs—like during certain points in your menstrual cycle or menopause—you might feel like your mental rhythm is off, leading to mood swings and brain fog.

Oestrogen isn't just about keeping your reproductive system in check—it also plays a big role in your mood and cognitive functions. When oestrogen levels are high, you're likely to feel happier and more balanced, thanks to its influence on serotonin, the brain's feel-good neurotransmitter. But when oestrogen dips, so can your mood and mental clarity, making those PMS moments feel all too real. On the flip side, too much oestrogen, particularly partnered with too little progesterone can cause all sorts of mayhem within the body leading to anxious or depressive moods or chronic illness such as endometriosis or adenomyosis. The key here, and with everything in life, is balance.

Hormones

Progesterone is the calming slow dancer, swaying gently to the soothing tunes of GABA, your brain's natural chill-out neurotransmitter. When progesterone is in the lead, you're likely to feel relaxed and at ease. But if progesterone stumbles, irritability and mood swings can take over, making you feel like the DJ just switched to a jarring techno beat.

Testosterone is the confident, slightly swaggering dancer who's all about spatial awareness and problem-solving. With testosterone in charge, you might find yourself breezing through tasks that require quick thinking and decisiveness. But if testosterone takes a backseat, you could feel less sharp, like you've suddenly forgotten the steps to a familiar dance.

Testosterone might be the hormone most often associated with men, but it's just as important for women. It's the hormone that gives you that extra boost of confidence, assertiveness, and mental sharpness. When levels are low, it can leave you feeling fatigued, irritable, and even a bit blue.

Hormonal Changes Throughout Life

As you move through life, your hormone levels will change, affecting your mood and cognitive functions differently at different stages. Understanding these changes is key to managing them and maintaining a balanced, positive outlook.

Managing Hormonal Impacts

The good news is that you can take steps to manage the impact of hormones on your mood and cognition. Nourishing your body with the right foods, moving your body in alignment with your cycle and daily energy cues and various other factors that we will discuss in depth in part II of this book are all crucial for keeping your hormones—and your mood—in check. By understanding how your hormones affect your mood and cognition, you can take control of your emotional and mental well-being, even when your hormones are fluctuating.

Cognition and Mood: The Hormonal Symphony

Now, we have established that hormones are little biochemical messengers, the unsung heroes (or sometimes more like villains) of our daily lives. While they're busy ensuring that our bodies run as a well-oiled machine, they're also conducting an elaborate symphony in our brains, determining how we think, feel, and react. Let's dive into how this all plays out:

If your emotions ever feel like a wild roller coaster ride, you can thank your hormones for that. Imagine them as the operators, sometimes speeding things up, sometimes slowing them down, and occasionally sending you into a loop-de-loop of emotions.

- **Premenstrual Syndrome (PMS)**: Right before your period, oestrogen and progesterone fluctuate which can create a disturbance in your mood regulation. This time of the month is typically associated with mood swings, irritability and anxiety, making you feel like your emotional rollercoaster has suddenly hit a sharp turn, and you're left holding on for dear life.

  What if these feelings were really trying to guide you to prioritise self-care, take rest, spend a little bit of time in isolation and sift through your own internal workings? You have the option to work WITH your body's wildy and wonderfully ingrained internal clock and take this cue to give yourself a break. Alone time can provide an opportunity to achieve a refreshing clarity on your own wants, needs and desires without the interruption of external influence that usually presides in our lives. When we listen to the whisper, our body doesn't have to shout.

- **Pregnancy and Postpartum**: Pregnancy can feel like an emotional high, with oestrogen and progesterone pumping up the good vibes. But after childbirth, these hormone levels drop faster than the stock market on a bad day, sometimes leading to the emotional lows of postpartum depression.

- **Menopause**: As oestrogen levels start to decline during menopause, the emotional rollercoaster might feel a bit more rickety, with mood swings, depression, and anxiety becoming more frequent riders.

Hormones don't just toy with your emotions; they're also the puppeteers behind your cognitive performance. When your hormones are in harmony, you might feel like a mental superhero, effortlessly conquering tasks and keeping everything in perfect order. But when they're out of whack, even the simplest of chores can feel like trying to solve a Rubik's Cube in the dark. We discussed mood, now let's take a closer look at how these key hormones play their part in your cognition:

When oestrogen is at its peak, you might find yourself breezing through tasks, with a memory sharper than a tack. It's like your brain has switched to high-definition mode, where everything is clear, vibrant, and in focus. However, when oestrogen levels dip, you might start misplacing your keys or struggling to remember names (more than usual), as if your brain has suddenly gone fuzzy and switched to low-res.

Cortisol, in small doses, is like the over-caffeinated colleague who helps you remember crucial details in stressful situations. It's there to boost your memory and get you through the tough times. If cortisol decides to hang around like an unwelcome guest, it can start to erode your mental sharpness, leaving you feeling like your brain is running on fumes and struggling to keep up.

Testosterone is the hormone that boosts your spatial abilities and problem-solving skills, like having a built-in GPS for navigating life's challenges. When testosterone is on your side, you can confidently chart your course through complex tasks. When testosterone levels drop, that once-clear mental map might start to look a little blurry, making it harder to find your way.

Progesterone, often overshadowed by its flashier counterparts, is the zen master of hormones. It works behind the scenes to keep your brain calm, collected, and clear-headed. When progesterone levels are steady, your mind feels serene, allowing you to focus and think clearly, even in the midst of chaos. When progesterone levels dip—perhaps due to stress, certain points in your menstrual cycle, or as a precursor to menopause—you might find yourself feeling mentally scattered, like your once-still pond has been disturbed by a sudden storm.

Progesterone's influence on the brain is deeply tied to its interaction with GABA (gamma-aminobutyric acid), the neurotransmitter responsible for calming the nervous system. When progesterone is abundant, it boosts GABA's soothing effects, helping you to feel relaxed

and mentally clear.
When progesterone takes a nosedive, it's as if GABA's calming influence is suddenly on vacation, leaving your mind more susceptible to anxiety, mood swings, and a general sense of mental clutter.
Understanding how these hormones influence your cognition can feel like cracking the code to your mental performance. By keeping them balanced—through proper nutrition, exercise, stress management, and sleep—you can ensure that they're working with you rather than against you. The next time you feel as if your brain is either soaring through tasks or trudging through molasses, remember: it's all part of the intricate hormonal dance happening within.

Maintaining a healthy hormonal balance doesn't require an advanced degree in biochemistry—just a few lifestyle tweaks can make a world of difference:

- **Nutrition**: Think of your nutrition as the fuel for your hormonal engine. Nutrient-rich foods, especially those packed with omega-3s, can help stabilise your mood and support cognitive function. It's like giving your brain premium fuel instead of regular unleaded.

- **Movement**: Regular physical activity is like a reset button for your hormones. It helps regulate cortisol levels, boosts endorphins, and keeps your brain firing on all cylinders.

- **Stress**: Techniques like meditation and yoga are the equivalent of giving your brain a spa day, helping to lower cortisol levels and reduce the negative impact of stress on your cognitive and emotional health.

Hormones

- **Sleep**: Never underestimate the power of a good night's sleep. Adequate rest is crucial for hormone regulation, mood stabilisation, and cognitive function. Think of sleep as the nightly maintenance your brain needs to stay in top form.

By taking these steps, you can ensure that your hormones are more of a supportive dance partner than an unruly guest at the party, keeping your mind sharp, your mood balanced, and your brain healthy for years to come. We will discuss these in more depth in Part II.

Trauma.

A quick important note:
It's often not the extreme cases of trauma that shape us the most, but rather the 'minor' day-to-day experiences that quietly pile up over a lifetime. These seemingly small events can weave their way into complex, subconscious beliefs that influence our choices and perceptions, requiring a combination of expert-level detective work and fearless self-awareness to decode and process.

Ignoring this work is essentially the same as letting your dog steer the car—adorable and mildly entertaining, yet absolutely destined for disaster.

An example of an everyday trauma might be a parent casually pointing out that you're 'getting a bit chubby' as a child. While seemingly harmless, repeated moments like this can plant seeds of insecurity and self-doubt that grow into deep-rooted beliefs, impacting how you view your body and self-worth for years to come.

Trauma

Let's cut to the chase—if you've got unresolved trauma lurking in the shadows, your nervous system might as well be playing a chaotic symphony, where the instruments are out of tune, and the conductor has gone missing. But don't worry, we're about to dive into how trauma impacts your body and what you can do to restore some much-needed harmony.

Bessel van der Kolk's seminal work, The Body Keeps the Score, provides key insights into this topic. It may take you on a bit of a rollercoaster—yes, it's a bit terrifying to learn just how deeply trauma can affect us, but it's also hopeful, like discovering that there's a way to disembark the ride safely. Van der Kolk has spent decades delving into the murky waters of trauma, leading to breakthroughs in neuroscience and psychology. His research underscores that trauma is more common than we'd like to admit; whether it's neglect, abuse, or any other traumatic event, understanding it is the first step toward healing.

First, let's discuss the almond shaped brain region located in the anterior portion of your temporal lobe, your amygdala. Imagine your amygdala as the world's most overzealous smoke detector, going off at the slightest hint of burnt toast. If you experience a traumatic event, the amygdala, your brain's alarm system, can become hypersensitive and overactive, triggering false alarms at every corner.

Meanwhile, your frontal lobes, the "watchtower" that usually steps in to say, "hey, it's just toast, not a house fire," start struggling to keep up. This leaves you in a constant state of alertness, which is as exhausting as it sounds. This prolonged state doesn't just wear down your mind—it takes a toll on your body too, manifesting as chronic pain, muscle tension, and even hormone-related issues like painful periods and gut problems. It's like your body is the stage, and trauma is the relentless director demanding an encore.

Unresolved trauma doesn't just pack its bags and leave after the event—until it is safely addressed, it sets up camp in your muscles, causing tension that can lead to spasms, back pain, migraines, and other forms of chronic pain. The good news? You can show it the door. Mindfulness practices such as yoga and meditation can help calm your nervous system, making it less likely that you'll be thrown into fight-or-flight mode at the slightest provocation. Working with a somatic therapist or trauma informed practitioner enables you to safely address the unresolved trauma that you are currently holding and once you find it, you can then begin to let it go.

Why is it critical to do this work and let go of your unresolved trauma? Trauma doesn't just trap you in the past—it keeps you from fully living in the present. Those lingering stress hormones keep replaying past defensive responses, making minor irritations feel like major threats, or leaving you feeling detached from life's significant events. Mastering your internal sensations and emotions is key to breaking free from this loop. Through neuroplasticity—your brain's ability to reorganise itself—you can transform these dysregulated patterns, helping you stay calm and focused, even when life tries to throw you off balance.

Triggers can feel debilitating and often, in my own experience, it can create a feeling of isolation. This is where holding strong and nurturing relationships can be an actual life saver. Let's not underestimate the power of a good hug. Positive relationships are like a security blanket for your nervous system, offering both physical and psychological protection. Traumatised individuals often find their footing again within the context of supportive relationships, where they can muster the bravery to face and process reality.

The sympathetic nervous system is the friend who's always ready to throw down at the slightest provocation, triggering your fight-or-flight response. Meanwhile, the parasympathetic nervous system (PSNS) is your zen master, coaxing you into relaxation once the threat has passed. By engaging in activities that activate the PSNS— meditation, deep breathing, yoga, spending time with friends or simply spending time in nature—you can lower stress, improve mood, and even give your immune system a little boost. It's like pressing your personal chill button. Sounds simple? It is.

Let's get one thing straight: self-care isn't just about bubble baths and scented candles (though those are nice too). For someone with PTSD, self-care means actively choosing safe relationships, practising mindful breathing, and working with a trauma-focused therapist. It's about creating an environment where you can heal, not just survive.

Trauma

When it comes to managing trauma, there's a veritable toolbox of therapies designed to help you process and heal from your experiences. Here's a peek at some of the most effective ones:

1. **EFT (Emotional Freedom Techniques)**: Imagine combining cognitive therapy with acupressure and you get EFT, or "tapping." By tapping on specific meridian points while focusing on traumatic memories, EFT can help balance the body's energy system, reduce stress, and improve emotional regulation.
   This process helps you to develop a safe internal environment, conducive to processing and releasing trauma.

2. **EMDR (Eye Movement Desensitization and Reprocessing)**: This therapy uses bilateral stimulation (like following a therapist's finger) to desensitise traumatic memories, helping you reprocess them into something less distressing.

3. **Shaking**: It sounds simple, but shaking can be a powerful way to release tension and trauma stored in the body. Animals do it instinctively after a stressful encounter, and humans can benefit from this natural stress reliever too.

4. **Dancing**: Movement therapy through dance helps you process emotions and connect with your body in a way that words sometimes can't. Plus, it's a mood booster that gets those endorphins flowing.

5. **Yoga**: Combining physical postures, breathwork, and meditation, yoga helps reduce stress, increase mindfulness, and improve overall physical health—making it a holistic approach to trauma therapy.

6. **Breath work**: Controlled breathing techniques, like diaphragmatic breathing, can activate the PSNS, reduce anxiety, and promote

self-awareness. This is one of the primary strategies that I implement with clients to create a safe internal foundation.

7. **Self-Compassion**: Practising self-compassion means treating yourself with the same kindness you'd offer a friend in need. It's about first identifying and then breaking the cycle of self-judgement and switching that inner critic to a voice of solace.

8. **Speaking to a Support Person/Group**: Sharing your experiences with a trusted friend, therapist, or support group can provide validation, build connections, and offer emotional release. It's a reminder that you don't have to go through this alone.

Self-criticism and judgement often stem from a primal need for external validation—something that once ensured our survival in a tribe but now leaves us vulnerable to pain. Practising grounding techniques can help you maintain calm amidst the chaos, and choosing to speak to yourself with compassion is a tangible way to foster self-love. This isn't about becoming a different, more "loveable" version of yourself for others—it's about being your own confidant, you are the one and only person that will reliably be with you every second of every day, it's your most important relationship, make it a good one.

If trauma is impacting your life, if you feel a little out of sorts, or if you are a human, 1 on 1 coaching with a trauma informed practitioner can help you set up a safe internal space, identify triggers, and release them in a supportive environment.

Trauma

How does trauma mess with your romance?

Think of trauma as that unwelcome guest at your romantic dinner—uninvited, yet determined to upend your evening. Left unaddressed, trauma can warp how you connect with others, making genuine, fulfilling relationships feel more like chasing a mirage. Instead of fostering closeness, you might build walls, mistrust shadows, and adopt survival strategies that do more harm than good. Trauma doesn't just mess with your head; it rewires your nervous system, making trust as elusive as a well-trained cat.

Trauma isn't just about what happened—it's also about what didn't. Those unmet needs, the love and security that were absent, leave a gaping void. This void doesn't just sit there quietly; it festers, influencing your thoughts, feelings, and interactions in ways that can be downright perplexing. It's less about the actual memories and more about how these experiences have become subconsciously ingrained, affecting your present-day responses.

Ever wonder why certain fears or beliefs pop up in your relationships? Chances are, they're echoes of past traumas. Trauma isn't about the event itself but how you process it, and no trauma is too small to matter. Unresolved trauma is the baggage you carry into every new relationship, leading to unhealthy behaviours that sabotage your chances at romance. When these wounds are left to fester, they don't just go away—they morph into patterns that confuse both you and your partner.

Ignoring unresolved wounds is like slapping a band-aid on a broken leg—ineffective and fundamentally disastrous. You might try to "suck it up," but these wounds will inevitably spill over into your relationships. Triggers from your past resurface, leading to emotional reactions that leave your partner scratching their head. For example, if you grew up with emotionally distant parents, something as simple as your partner coming home late might feel like a repeat performance of abandonment.

Even if your partner has the best intentions, trauma skews your perception, making you see threats where there are none. You might struggle to express your worth, resulting in a relationship where unresolved trauma becomes the lens through which you view the world.

- **Hot and Cold Dynamics**: One minute, you're all in, and the next, you're pulling back. This push-pull creates tension and trust issues.
- **Bonding Over Shared Trauma**: While it's comforting to connect over similar wounds, this often leads to unhealthy dynamics where you end up trying to "save" each other—a recipe for disaster.
- **Perfectionism**: Growing up in a critical or invalidating environment might push you to seek perfection in yourself or your relationships, leading to workaholism, extreme exercise, or disordered eating as you strive to overcompensate for feelings of inadequacy.
- **Avoiding Healing**: Some use relationships as a distraction, hopping from partner to partner to avoid facing their own pain.
- **Seeking External Validation**: When you try to fill a self-love void with romantic relationships, you might overlook red flags, leading to unfulfilling connections.

Trauma

If you're stuck in these patterns, it's crucial to know that healing is possible—and you don't have to do it alone. Working with a trauma-informed practitioner can provide the support you need to begin healing these maladaptive behaviours. Rediscover your sense of self, independence, and autonomy, and take a closer look at how your early experiences have shaped your relationships.

Healing isn't a straight path, and it doesn't happen overnight. It can feel lonely, and the temptation to fast-forward through the process is strong. But remember, there's no such thing as "normal." Everyone has their baggage, and the key is learning how to manage yours while you work through it.

- **Respect Boundaries**: Before unloading your trauma on someone, make sure they're in a place to handle it. Boundaries are vital for both of you.
- **Seek Professional Help**: Trauma-informed professionals can relieve some of the burden from your personal relationships, allowing you to heal in a safe environment.
- **Embrace Self-Compassion**: I have said it before and I will say it again, self-compassion can change your life. Accepting yourself as you are now is the first step toward growth and change.
  Self-compassion is your best ally in this journey.
- **Implement Your Own Boundaries**: Setting boundaries might feel daunting, but it's absolutely essential. Respecting yourself helps others respect you, too.
  Here's a reassuring truth: you're not losing anything worth keeping by setting boundaries. The only people who get irritated by your boundaries are the ones who intended to overstep them. When

someone drops out of your life because of your boundaries, it creates a space—an opportunity to fill that gap with something, or someone, better.

In my own journey, I've faced countless internal hurdles that made setting boundaries feel nearly impossible—my lack of self-worth, a deep-seated fear of abandonment (as if someone's presence, or lack there of, could define my value), and the gnawing anxiety that someone might respond in a way that threatened my safety. Healing from these patterns didn't happen overnight, and it's still an ongoing process that takes a lot of courage and brutally honest self-reflection. I had to break down old beliefs and release the self-blame that I once clung to as a form of control, but that ultimately fuelled self-sabotage and pain. This work was supported by a therapist I learned to trust over time, and it led to tears, emotional unearthing, and facing truths I'd long avoided. Working through the pain—going through the emotional tunnel—is the only way to reach the light on the other side. Yes, it's tough, but trust me: it makes the rest of your life feel lighter, sweeter, and far more manageable.

Let me add this: it's ok to take your time with this work.
I couldn't start immediately after significant trauma; it took years for me to build the internal and external safety I needed—a stable home, a steady income, supportive relationships, a balanced life, and solid emotional grounding. Dealing and healing are two ends of a spectrum, and both are necessary at different points in your life. Sometimes, you just need to focus on dealing until you're ready to truly heal.

Pause here for a moment.

Take a breath.

We are covering a lot of dense information and it is important to be gentle with yourself in your expectation of learning and retaining all of this in one hit.

Just sit for a second and congratulate yourself on how far you have come. You are well on your way to hitting 'Nervous System and Trauma Mastermind' status. GO you!

Trauma

... still pausing...

... OK ready.

Trauma

Detoxing from your Ex

"But how do I let go?". We all have people, habits, and beliefs that we allow into our inner sanctuary when we know deep down that they not only don't benefit us, but actively limit, restrict, or cloud our judgement on a daily basis. Why? Because you my love are human.

This is part of the journey, navigating the wild waters of life and consciously deciding which parts you want to integrate and which parts you don't. This will eb and flow over time, what serves the person you are and the goals you have now probably won't be the exact same in 10 years, 5 years, 1 year, 2 months or possibly even an hour from now. One moment you feel like laying down on the couch to rest and the next you feel that you need fresh air and sunshine - both serve a purpose, at different points in time.

When it is time to let something go, this can be challenging due to the neural circuits in your brain having practised this pathway so many times that it has now become the favoured pathway of choice. A practised habit feels to your brain like a sunset stroll on the beach with your beloved holding your hand, and a new habit feels like a midnight trek up a cold cliff with no torchlight.

Focus on peace, not uncertainty: You're choosing to let go because it no longer activates a sense of peacefulness within yourself or your life. Often letting go of something feels like a loss, but you can flip that script to focus on the peace that you are gaining, rather than the thing you are losing.

Trauma

Your energy is valuable: Think of how much energy you've been investing in trying to "just make it work." Every time you feel the urge to repeat this pattern, remind yourself that you deserve to invest that energy back into yourself, your goals, and the people, habits and beliefs that actively contribute to your well-being. Relentlessly surround yourself with what increases your energy and capacity, if something is draining it - remind yourself, "I deserve better".

If we are talking specifically about letting go of a person - Reclaim control: Instead of reaching out, remind yourself that by not doing so, you're taking control of the situation. You're no longer waiting for this person to give you clarity—you're creating your own. We think that by reaching out, we will receive a sense of clarity via the reply of the person on the other end. The truth is, you already know the answer.

Ask yourself: Will this bring me what I want? If you feel tempted to reconnect or repeat, ask if doing so will actually help you feel fulfilled, or if it's just a temporary way to soothe discomfort. The long-term clarity and peace will outweigh the short-term relief.

Focus on closure, not continuation: Remind your brain that by letting go, you're closing a chapter that wasn't bringing you the emotional safety and connection you deserve. Every step away from it is a step toward something better.

The 'Toxic' Cleanse: When the brain detoxes from a breakup, it's not unlike kicking a bad habit—except this habit wore your favourite cologne and sent sweet texts late at night. Love, after all, is like the finest vintage wine for the brain, intoxicating it with dopamine and oxytocin until you're tipsy with connection. So, when the relationship unceremoniously ends, the brain is left scrambling for another glass, wandering around the emotional bar like a heartbroken regular who's been cut off. Cue the withdrawal: sudden mood swings, tidal waves of sadness, and that infamous brain fog, where even remembering to water your plants feels like solving quantum physics.

But, as with any good detox, there comes a moment when the brain starts to adjust. Slowly but surely, the mental clutter clears, and the neurotransmitters begin to shuffle back to their rightful places, like employees returning after a long holiday, a little rusty but ready to work. The brain, much like a house in need of renovation, starts stripping away those old, creaky neural pathways that once revolved around your ex. The scaffolding goes up, and before you know it, new connections are being built—ones that don't involve late-night tears or stalking their Instagram.

As time goes on, clarity arrives like a long-awaited sunrise after a storm. You stop seeing the relationship through the rose-tinted glasses of nostalgia and start recognising it for the maze it often was. The brain, now free from its chemical addiction, steps out of the wreckage and into the fresh air, ready to embrace new adventures, wiser and lighter for having endured the detox. Like any great comeback story, you emerge from the rubble—sipping a metaphorical green juice, of course—ready to take on life without the chains of the past holding you back.
Letting go of someone or something you love, yet know is no longer serving you, might just be one of the hardest feats of human endurance. Trust me, I'm right there with you. In fact, I just re-read this chapter for myself because, if I'm being honest, I need these reminders as much as anyone. Mastering the art of release isn't a one-time thing—it's a delicate dance of practice, patience, and a bucketload of self

compassion. As you navigate this, be kind to yourself. You deserve that love and tenderness more than anyone.
I believe in you—and you should too.

3 tangible strategies to apply here:

1. Ask yourself: What do I need to learn from this, to let it go?
I find physically writing this out in a journal to be the most effective method.

2. Swap don't stop: Trying to just 'stop thinking' is the same as trying to just, not require oxygen anymore… it doesn't really work like that. Instead, you can refocus your mind on a healthier thought process / question: How can I love myself better?

3. Consciously choose your hard… Ask yourself, which "hard" do I want? Because, truth be told, both roads—the one where you stay and the one where you go—are challenging. I've been there. In fact, I recently cut things off with someone I really enjoyed spending time with. Our dates were always fun, filled with delicious dinners and great conversations. We got along so well that we could talk for hours, but when my grandfather passed away, I texted him and… crickets. Three days passed before he responded. That moment laid bare the lack of depth between us, yet the good times were so intoxicating that I kept pushing the nagging feeling aside.

Although it felt somewhat exciting and alluring, it left me feeling hollow and uneasy. Some days I left his company feeling on top of the world; other times, I wasn't sure if he was already halfway out the door. The attention was inconsistent, like a tap dripping unpredictably and I never knew if it would pour or run dry. It was thrilling, sure—like a hit of something addictive—but the comedown was brutal. I was choosing the hard of unpredictable highs and inevitable lows, hoping it would get better when in fact, it was unravelling before my eyes.

Then, after sending a particularly vulnerable message and watching it collect dust for a week, I finally admitted it to myself: I had to walk away. It wasn't easy. I didn't want to, but I knew I had been accepting far less than I deserved because I feared the withdrawal. Yet, I made the choice to switch my "hard." I decided that the temporary pain of withdrawal, with the promise of long-term peace and the lesson to trust my gut in the future, was better than the constant cycle of waiting for crumbs of affection from someone who wasn't truly invested.

Ending things was... very shitty. For weeks, all I wanted was to reach out—ok, confession time, in a weak moment, I did and he didn't respond, which, in hindsight, was the best gift that he could've given me.
Along the way, I implemented a new strategy: every time he crept into my thoughts, I asked myself, "Did this relationship bring me peace?" (Spoiler alert: the answer is no).

With this strategy in place, I slowly stopped romanticising the fun moments and began valuing myself enough to stop settling for someone that showed he didn't really value me.

To do this work, I have to be relentlessly and courageously curious with myself. It means creating an internal dialogue that's safe, non-judgemental, and compassionate—a space where even the most hidden parts of me feel welcome to surface. I have to slow down, sit in stillness, and allow myself the time to listen, really listen, to what's beneath the surface.

Trauma

Sometimes, this looks like revisiting a childhood memory and rewriting the narrative. Other times, it's about completing the emotional process of a trauma that was left unfinished. It's not easy, but it's essential work—because until we make space to truly tap into ourselves, those unhealed parts will continue to influence our present in ways we don't always understand.

If you choose to embark on your own journey of self-discovery and healing, please remember: you don't have to do it alone. Whether it's me or another trauma-informed practitioner you feel drawn to, there are people ready to support you, to guide you, and to ensure your journey is safe, empowering, and transformative. Healing isn't something you have to face in isolation—it's something you're meant to feel held through.

Reminders:

1. My life functions to the standard that I allow.

2. If I want to let go, I have to fall madly in love with that part of myself that is holding on.

3. What someone else values and their capacity for this relationship is not a reflection on me or my worth, it is a reflection of their past, their belief systems (conscious and subconscious) and what works for them.

Think With Your Gut.

Think With Your Gut

"Trust your gut" isn't just wise advice for decision-making; it's also a crucial reminder of how your gut health plays a pivotal role in regulating hormones. The gut, often referred to as the "second brain," is teeming with neurotransmitters and neurons, making the gut-brain connection a fundamental aspect of your overall well-being.

The Gut as a Neurotransmitter Powerhouse

Your gut is a major producer of neurotransmitters, surpassing even the brain in some respects. It produces approximately 90% of the body's serotonin—often dubbed the "feel-good" neurotransmitter—critical for mood regulation, anxiety control, and emotional stability.

- **Serotonin**: Beyond its role in mood regulation, serotonin influences gut motility (the movement of the digestive tract) and the function of smooth muscles. Imbalances in serotonin can lead to digestive issues like irritable bowel syndrome (IBS) and destabilise your mood.
- **Dopamine**: While dopamine is typically associated with the brain, it's also produced in the gut, playing a role in regulating movement, memory, the pleasurable reward motivation and emotional responses.

The Gut-Brain Axis: A Constant Dialogue

The gut-brain axis is a two-way communication system between your central nervous system (CNS) and the enteric nervous system (ENS) within your gastrointestinal tract. This axis facilitates constant dialogue between your brain and gut, impacting everything from digestion to mood.

- **Vagus Nerve**: We have spoken about this in length in the previous chapter. Your vagus nerve acts as the primary highway connecting the gut and brain, it plays a crucial role in modulating inflammation, stress responses, and digestion.
- **Microbiota**: The trillions of microbes residing in your gut, collectively known as the microbiota, are key players in this communication. A balanced microbiota produces short-chain fatty acids (SCFAs) that influence brain function and neurotransmitter production.

How Gut Health Influences Hormones

1. **Cortisol and Stress Response:**
   Your gut microbiota directly influences your body's stress response. An imbalance in gut bacteria (dysbiosis) can lead to increased cortisol production—the infamous stress hormone. As you now know, elevated cortisol can wreak havoc on sleep, mood, and menstrual cycles.

2. **Oestrogen Metabolism:**
   Gut bacteria are instrumental in metabolising and recycling oestrogen. Specific bacteria produce an enzyme called beta-glucuronidase (you don't really need to remember that), which helps reabsorb oestrogen from the gut into the bloodstream. An imbalance can result in either oestrogen dominance or deficiency, affecting menstrual health, mood and lead to hormonal disorders such as adenomyosis and impact symptoms of endometriosis.

3. **Thyroid Function:**
   Your gut plays a role in converting inactive thyroid hormone (T4) into its active form (T3). A healthy gut ensures efficient conversion

and absorption of thyroid hormones, which are vital for metabolism, energy levels, and overall hormonal balance.

4. **Insulin Sensitivity and Blood Sugar Regulation:**
   Gut health also impacts insulin sensitivity and blood sugar regulation. Dysbiosis can lead to insulin resistance, contributing to conditions like PCOS (Polycystic Ovary Syndrome) and disrupting overall hormonal balance.

Practical Tips for Nurturing Gut Health

1. **Nutrition**: Our bodies are all beautifully unique and different, and it is vital to understand that what works for one person may not work for another. Below is a few suggestions that are safe for you to experiment with, to see how it feels in your own body.

- **Prebiotics**: Incorporate foods like garlic, onions, leeks, asparagus, and bananas to feed the beneficial bacteria in your gut.
- **Probiotics**: Include fermented foods such as yoghurt, kefir, sauerkraut, kimchi, and kombucha to introduce beneficial bacteria.
- **Fibre**: Maintain a diet rich in fibre from vegetables, fruits, legumes, and whole grains to support healthy digestion and nourish your gut microbiota.

2. **Hydration**: Drinking plenty of filtered water helps maintain the mucosal lining of your intestines and supports the balance of beneficial bacteria.

3. **Stress**: Engage in practices such as breathwork, meditation, and yoga to help cope with stress and its negative impact on gut health. This may seem to be one of the more elusive suggestions that are discussed in this book yet it is possibly the most important. A quick fix can happen through changing nutrition and drinking more water but implementing mindfulness through the practices discussed above will create the most profound long term change in your life.

4. **Regular Exercise**: Physical activity promotes healthy gut motility and reduces stress, contributing to a balanced gut microbiota.

5. **Sleep**: Prioritise quality sleep—aim for 7-9 hours of uninterrupted sleep each night to maintain gut health. We will elaborate on the impact of sleep in Part II of this book.

Understanding the gut's impact on hormonal balance is like tuning into a symphony where every section must play in harmony. By nurturing your gut health, you support the delicate interplay of neurotransmitters and hormones, leading to improved mood, energy levels, and overall well-being. Next time you're told to "trust your gut," remember—it's not just good advice for your mind but for your body as well.

Methylation.

Methylation

Methylation is a critical biochemical process happening billions of times each day in every cell of your body. Think of it as a kind of "biological switch," where a small molecular group made up of one carbon and three hydrogen atoms (a "methyl group") is transferred to DNA, proteins, or neurotransmitters. This tiny switch has a profound impact on numerous body functions, including gene expression, detoxification, hormone regulation, and neurotransmitter production. Let's break down how methylation influences these areas and why it's crucial for mental and physical health.

1. Gene Expression: Methylation plays a major role in turning genes "on" or "off." By adding a methyl group to DNA, the body can silence or activate specific genes. This process is not just about preventing or allowing gene activity—it's about controlling when and how much of a gene's instructions are used. For instance, methylation helps to keep genes in check that, when overly active, could contribute to conditions such as cancer.
By "bookmarking" sections of our DNA, methylation helps our cells differentiate, develop, and function according to their intended roles.

2. Detoxification: Our bodies encounter toxins daily—from pollutants in the air to chemicals in our food. Methylation is essential in detoxifying these compounds, particularly by processing harmful substances through the liver. This "methylation detox" allows the body to clear out toxins efficiently, supporting everything from brain function to cellular health. Impaired methylation can lead to toxin build-up, which, over time, may result in fatigue, inflammation, and even disease.

3. Neurotransmitter Production: Methylation is crucial for the production and regulation of neurotransmitters, such as serotonin, dopamine, adrenaline, and norepinephrine—chemicals that influence mood, focus, sleep, and overall mental well-being. For example:

- **Serotonin and Melatonin:**
  Methylation helps convert tryptophan to 5-HTP, the precursor to serotonin, a neurotransmitter essential for mood balance. It also helps convert serotonin into melatonin, our sleep-regulating hormone.

- **Dopamine and Adrenaline:**
  Methylation assists in transporting dopamine, norepinephrine, and adrenaline across neural pathways. It also aids in converting norepinephrine into adrenaline, essential for focus and attention. The proper functioning of these neurotransmitters helps us manage stress, feel balanced, and maintain mental clarity. If methylation is disrupted, however, the production of these mood-regulating chemicals can suffer, potentially leading to feelings of anxiety, depression, or mental fatigue.

4. Hormone Regulation

Hormones, the body's messengers, play a role in everything from energy levels to reproductive health. Methylation helps regulate hormones by breaking down excess levels of certain hormones, such as estrogen. An imbalance in methylation can lead to hormone fluctuations, contributing to mood swings, energy dips, and even chronic conditions like hormone-related cancers.

5. The Role of Environmental and Lifestyle Factors in Methylation

Methylation doesn't happen in isolation; it's influenced by various factors like diet, stress, environmental toxins, and even genetics. Poor diet, high in processed foods and low in essential nutrients, can impair methylation. Nutrients like folate, B12, B6, riboflavin (B2), magnesium, and zinc are crucial for optimal methylation. Folate, for instance, is essential for producing methyl donors, compounds that donate methyl groups in the methylation process.

- **Oxidative Stress:** Exposure to environmental toxins and free radicals can increase oxidative stress, which in turn disrupts methylation. Maintaining a diet rich in antioxidants can help balance oxidative stress and support methylation.

- **Genetic Variants:** Certain gene variations, such as the MTHFR gene mutation, can impact the body's ability to produce enzymes needed for methylation. This genetic variation might result in slower methylation, which can lead to elevated homocysteine levels (a risk factor for cardiovascular and cognitive issues).

6. Impact on Mental Health and Well-being

Because methylation influences neurotransmitter production, it has a profound impact on mental health. For instance, low levels of methylation-related nutrients, like B vitamins and magnesium, are often associated with mood disorders. Methylation regulates dopamine and serotonin, which can affect our resilience to stress and ability to experience pleasure. A poorly functioning methylation cycle may be associated with issues like depression, anxiety, difficulty focusing, and chronic fatigue.

Methylation

Supporting Healthy Methylation Through Lifestyle Choices

- **Nutrition:** Leafy greens, legumes, nuts, seeds, and lean proteins are rich in folate, B vitamins, and other essential nutrients that fuel the methylation process.

- **Avoid Toxins:** Limiting exposure to toxins, such as alcohol, tobacco, and environmental pollutants, helps to prevent disruptions in methylation.

- **Regular Exercise:** Physical activity promotes antioxidant production, which balances oxidative stress, protecting the methylation cycle from disruption.

Methylation is a small but mighty process that keeps many of our body's functions in balance. It's essential for mental and physical health, from gene expression and detoxification to neurotransmitter production and hormone regulation. Disruptions in methylation can have wide-ranging effects on health, including mood instability, cognitive challenges, and hormone imbalances. By understanding and supporting methylation, we can make choices that promote long-term well-being, keeping our bodies and minds balanced and functioning at their best.

Somatic Stress.

Somatic Stress

When Stress Manifests in the Body

Somatic stress might sound like a term plucked from a medical textbook, but it's essentially your body's dramatic way of spilling the tea about your inner turmoil. This concept highlights how psychological stress can stage a coup in your body, giving rise to tangible physical symptoms that can affect various bodily systems.

Buckle up, we are about to break down what somatic stress entails, its triggers, common signs, and how best to manage it.

What is Somatic Stress?

Imagine somatic stress as your body's melodramatic moment – it's when emotional or psychological stress decides to wear a neon sign, manifesting as physical symptoms. The term "somatic" comes from the Greek word "soma," meaning body. So, rather than stress playing mind games, somatic stress takes the runway in the form of physical discomfort or pain, often without an obvious medical cause.

Several factors are behind somatic stress's grand entrance, including:

1. **Chronic Stress:** Think of this like an unending group chat full of drama – prolonged exposure to stressful situations keeps your body's stress response in constant overdrive, eventually spilling into physical symptoms.

2. **Traumatic Events:** As we have discussed, past traumatic experiences can lurk in the shadows, only to subconsciously manifest as physical symptoms later – a bit like a ghosted texter suddenly resurfacing.

3. **Anxiety Disorders**: Generalised anxiety, panic disorders, and other anxiety-related conditions can come with a suitcase full of somatic baggage.

4. **Psychosocial Factors**: Interpersonal conflicts, work-related stress, and major life changes can all ignite somatic stress. Imagine these as those moments in life when your phone battery dies just as you're about to win an argument.

Common Symptoms of Somatic Stress

Somatic stress is like having your phone on vibrate – your body is constantly buzzing and mimicking symptoms of physical illness to try and get your attention. Common symptoms include:

1. **Muscle Tension and Pain**: Persistent muscle tightness, particularly in the neck, shoulders, and back. Tension headaches or migraines also love to RSVP.

2. **Gastrointestinal Issues**: Stomachaches, bloating, diarrhoea, or constipation. IBS, anyone?

3. **Cardiovascular Symptoms**: Palpitations, chest pain, or a feeling of tightness in the chest; it's like your heart's having an impromptu dance party without an invite. Increased heart rate and elevated blood pressure can join the mix as well.

4. **Respiratory Problems**: Shortness of breath or hyperventilation—a bit like that feeling when you spot your ex's name in your notifications. A tightness in the throat or chest might also drop by.

5. **Sleep Disturbances**: Insomnia, restless sleep, or constant wake-ups, as if your alarm clock has developed a cruel sense of humour. Night sweats or nightmares can make guest appearances too.

6. **Skin Reactions**: Rashes, hives, or unexplained itching, akin to a social media breakout. Your skin decides to turn into a drama queen, often worsening conditions like eczema or psoriasis.

7. **Fatigue and Weakness**: Persistent tiredness that refuses to leave even after that extra shot of espresso. Generalised weakness or a lack of energy makes it feel like your body's on low power mode.

8. **Reproductive System Issues**: Menstrual irregularities, such as missed periods or severe PMS—your body's way of throwing a tantrum. Also, a lowered libido or sexual dysfunction might pop up like an unwelcome DM.

Managing somatic stress involves addressing both the physical symptoms and the drama brewing underneath.
Strategies may include:

1. **Mind-Body Practices**:

- Mindfulness Meditation: Think of this as swiping left on negativity and matching with relaxation. It helps reduce overall stress and improve body awareness.
- Yoga: A perfect blend of physical movement and mindfulness to ease muscle tension and nurture relaxation. Downward dog, anyone?
- Tai Chi and Qigong: These gentle martial arts focus on fluid movements and deep breathing—your personal slow-mo filter for stress relief.

2. **Therapy and Counselling**:

- Cognitive Behavioural Therapy (CBT): This helps kick those pesky stress-related thought patterns to the curb. Think of this as digging up the dirt, it may not clear it out on its own but it can be helpful in deciphering what needs to be addressed.
- Somatic Therapy: An essential in somatic healing, focuses on the mind-body connection, helping to release stored tension and trauma—consider it a mental and physical detox.

3. **Physical Activity**:

- Regular exercise can lower stress hormones and elevate your mood—a little like finding a hidden stash of chocolate. Activities such as walking, swimming, or cycling can be particularly beneficial.

4. **Relaxation Techniques**:

- Deep Breathing: Engages the parasympathetic nervous system, promoting relaxation—imagine it as downloading a chillout playlist for your body.
- Progressive Muscle Relaxation: Involves tensing and then relaxing different muscle groups. Think of it as your body doing a series of stretch and release yoga poses.

5. **Healthy Lifestyle Choices**:

- Maintain a balanced diet rich in nutrients that support stress management. Like swapping fast food for a gourmet home-cooked meal.

- Ensure adequate hydration and limit caffeine and alcohol intake. Consider it upgrading from cheap instant coffee to premier organic brew.
- Prioritise sleep and establish a consistent sleep routine—think of it as setting your phone to 'Do Not Disturb' mode for your body.

6. **Support Systems**: Lean on friends, family, or support groups. Sharing your experiences is like having a squad to back you up during a group chat meltdown.

Somatic stress is a vivid reminder of how deeply intertwined our minds and bodies are. Recognising the symptoms and underlying causes of somatic stress is the first step towards taming this dramatic diva. By adopting a holistic approach that addresses both physical and psychological aspects, you can better navigate the tricky terrain of somatic stress and improve your overall well-being. The next time you feel a tension headache creeping in after a long, stressful day, remember—your body's just putting on a performance, signalling it's time to take a well-deserved break, both literally and figuratively.

Your Cycle.

Your Cycle

Menstruation: that charming monthly event when your uterus decides it's time for a little redecorating by shedding its lining. This process is orchestrated by a hormonal symphony conducted by your hypothalamus, pituitary gland, and ovaries. The menstrual cycle is divided into two acts: the follicular (or proliferative) phase and the luteal (or secretory) phase. The average cycle lasts 28 days, but anything from 25 to 30 days is perfectly normal. If your cycle is shorter than 21 days, welcome to the "polymenorrhea" club, and if it stretches beyond 35 days, you've entered the realm of "oligomenorrhea" – sounds posh, doesn't it?

In a typical month, you'll lose about 30 mL of blood. Go beyond 80 mL, and your body's truly testing your patience. The menstrual cycle tends to be erratic during life's bookends—menarche (your first period) and menopause—thanks to irregular ovulation and follicle development.

Follicular Phase: The follicular phase kicks off on day one of your period and sets the stage until ovulation. Think of it as your body's spring cleaning session, clearing out the old to make way for the new. This phase is marked by a lower basal body temperature and the growth of ovarian follicles, much like contestants getting ready in a reality show makeover episode. As the old hormone production wanes, follicle-stimulating hormone (FSH) rises to recruit a fresh crop of ovarian follicles. One lucky follicle gets selected to take the centre stage and mature, while oestrogen and inhibin B keep FSH from overdoing it. FSH activates aromatase enzymes in granulosa cells to convert androgens to oestrogen, creating a nurturing environment for the top follicle.

Your Cycle

Ovulation: Think of ovulation as the much-anticipated fashion show where the selected follicle finally takes its catwalk moment. This typically happens 10-12 hours after the LH (luteinizing hormone) peak, triggered by a big surge of oestrogen. The LH spike acts as the backstage crew, setting off a chain of events that leads to the egg's release. Picture the dominant follicle, now mature and over 15mm in diameter, taking the spotlight. The LH surge not only prompts ovulation but also kicks off progesterone production and the final preparation of the egg for its next journey.

The Luteal Phase: If the follicular phase is the spring clean and ovulation is the grand debut, the luteal phase is the cosy after-party. This phase, typically a steady 14 days, follows ovulation. Picture the granulosa cells that missed their chance to release the egg transforming into the corpus luteum, the event planner of your cycle, ensuring everything's set for a potential pregnancy. The corpus luteum secretes progesterone to prepare the endometrium, your body's VIP lounge, for a potential VIP guest—a fertilised egg. Around 8-9 days after ovulation, the phase reaches peak cosiness with maximum vascularisation, making the endometrium a plush, ready-for-implantation lining.
If pregnancy doesn't happen, the corpus luteum retires, turning into the corpus albicans, as progesterone and oestrogen levels fall, making way for the next cycle.

Oestrogen: Oestrogen, the star performer, has two main acts during your cycle: one in the mid-follicular phase and one in the mid-luteal phase. Its levels rise, fall, rise again, and then fall at the end of the cycle, like the riveting plot twists in your favourite binge-worthy series. When it's up, oestrogen prepares the endometrium and enhances your mood and energy levels. When it drops, it signals the end of the cycle, wrapping up the season and setting the stage for the next.

Oestrogen Dominance: Sometimes, the script goes off-track. When oestrogen takes centre stage for too long, the scene can get chaotic. Known as oestrogen dominance, this can lead to a suite of symptoms including weight gain, tender breasts, fibrocystic breasts, irregular or heavy periods, mood swings, decreased libido, headaches, hair loss, cold extremities, memory issues, insomnia, and fatigue. The challenge here is rebalancing the cast, ensuring oestrogen doesn't overshadow its co-stars. For a treasure trove of insights and tips on managing these symptoms, check out the plethora of blogs on Unprocessedapp.com

Endometrium: The endometrium is the unsung hero of your cycle, constantly working behind the scenes. Under the influence of oestrogen, it thickens to create a lush, inviting environment. Post-ovulation, progesterone takes over, further modifying the endometrium , transforming it into a plush, comfy cushion ready for potential implantation. If there's no pregnancy, the endometrium gets the memo and begins its gentle exit strategy. Think of this phase as the cleanup crew, guided by prostaglandins, that tidies up the venue, leading to menstruation where the endometrial lining is shed—preparing for the next grand event.

Hormonal Roller Coaster: At the end of your cycle, as oestrogen and progesterone levels plunge, the corpus luteum (our event planner) disbands. This drop triggers the release of prostaglandins, the contract-and-cleanup crew that induces uterine contractions, leading to the endometrial lining's shedding –
effectively pressing 'reset' for the next cycle.

Your Cycle

Cervix and Vagina: In our cycle's theatrical production, the cervix and vagina play vital supporting roles. Cervical mucus, the scene-changing crew, adapts in consistency and quantity throughout the cycle. Post-menstruation, it's scant and thick, but as ovulation approaches, it becomes clear and copious, like rolling out the red carpet for the egg. Post-ovulation, it thickens again, providing a snug security detail for any potential VIP guests.
Your vaginal cells also shift gears, reflecting these hormonal changes, and adapting to maintain a healthy, balanced environment.

The Brain and the Menstrual Cycle: As if this hormonal ballet wasn't enough, your menstrual cycle also choreographs subtle changes in your brain structure and function. It's like having a hidden playlist that sets the tempo for different acts of your day. Research suggests that while women often excel in verbal and memory tasks, men tend to outperform in spatial tasks. PMS, which affects up to 75% of women, can turn this delicate dance into a dramatic number, complete with mood swings, fatigue, and food cravings.
Studies show that brain activity varies with the menstrual cycle, affecting cognitive tasks and emotional responses, making it clear that your mind and body are in constant, intricate dialogue.

Embrace Compassion: Understanding the menstrual cycle and its hormonal influences can help you navigate its complexities with a touch of humour and a lot of empathy. Whether you're dealing with irregular periods, PMS, or oestrogen dominance, knowledge is power—and the first step to healing is meeting yourself with compassion and understanding that your body is truly working for you, not against you.

Your Cycle

Exercise: Moving with Your Cycle

- **Follicular Phase**: Really listen to your body in the first week of your cycle and opt for gentle practices. As you gain energy coming into the second week, you may feel inspired to consciously increase your training regime.
- **Ovulation (Mid-Cycle)**: This is peak energy for most girlies, however for some, mid-cycle can be a time of pain and discomfort, particularly for my oestrogen dominant girls. Be gentle with yourself, listen to your body and opt for rest when you feel called to. At this time, a cheeky sauna may be the perfect way to sweat without exacerbating any pain from an inflamed endometrium.
- **Luteal Phase (Post-Ovulation to Menstruation)**: Energy tends to wane. Stick to moderate exercises such as yoga, pilates, or light cardio. Listen to your body—it's completely fine to ease up.
- **Menstrual Phase**: Overlapping with the early stage of the Follicular phase. Focus on gentle movements such as stretching, walking, or restorative yoga. This is the time for self-care, not pushing limits.

Nutrition: Eating with Your Cycle

- **Follicular Phase**: Embrace fresh, vibrant foods rich in antioxidants (think berries, leafy greens).
  Protein and healthy fats are your buddies.
- **Ovulation**: Your metabolism is firing on all cylinders.
  Fuel it with nutrient-dense foods like lean proteins, whole grains, and plenty of veggies.

Your Cycle

- **Luteal Phase**: Cravings might spike. Balance your blood sugar with complex carbs, fibre, and protein. Magnesium-rich foods (nuts, seeds, dark chocolate) can help curb cravings.

- **Menstrual Phase**: Iron-rich foods (red meat, spinach) are essential to replenish lost stores. Stay hydrated and include anti-inflammatory foods like turmeric and ginger.

Structuring Your Tasks and Schedule

- **Follicular Phase**: Use your high energy for brainstorming, planning, and tackling challenging tasks.

- **Ovulation**: Your communication skills peak. Schedule important meetings, presentations, and social events during this time.

- **Luteal Phase**: Shift towards detail-oriented tasks and wrap up projects. Prioritise self-care and rest.

- **Menstrual Phase**: Reflect and review. Use this time for less intensive tasks like strategic thinking or planning for the next cycle.
  Take stock of your life, journal, anything to create space for yourself my honey.

What You Put In Your Mouth...

What You Put In Your Mouth...

Touching on Food

I'm not going to dwell too long on what you put in your mouth... and get your mind out of the gutter, I'm talking about food and drinks here! Let's briefly chat about how coffee and alcohol influence your nervous system. I won't dictate what's right for your body; only you can decide that by paying attention to how different foods make you feel, and maybe getting some blood tests or hormone and gut microbiome tests along the way.

I've personally experimented with various diets—vegan, vegetarian, ketogenic, calorie restriction, fasting, you name it. Through all of these, I've settled on two guiding principles:

1. A mostly unprocessed, whole food diet. Though, a cheeky croissant here and there is always welcome!

2. Swap, don't stop.

Intuitive Eating... But How?

1: Prioritise whole foods: This will allow your body to regulate its true cravings, free from artificial dopamine-fuelled sugar urges.

2. Breathe: Regulating your nervous system also decreases dopamine fuelled cravings.

3. Pay Attention: Take note of how different foods make you feel.

4. Eat Slowly and Chew Your Food: Digestion begins in your mouth - Savour each bite, giving your brain time to catch up with your stomach.

Side Note About Inflammation

Magnesium: Like a calming whisper to your muscles and nerves, magnesium reduces inflammation, improves sleep, and regulates blood sugar levels. Find it in leafy greens, nuts, seeds, and whole grains.

Celery Juice: Beyond Instagram trends, celery juice is packed with antioxidants and anti-inflammatory properties. It helps flush out toxins and supports digestion. A morning glass can be refreshing and clean your gut, all at once! We love efficiency.

Ginger Tea: My personal daily ritual. Ginger is a powerhouse of anti-inflammatory benefits. It soothes the digestive system, reduces muscle pain, and can even tackle morning sickness. Grate fresh ginger into a tea infuser and let it steep—it's like a warm hug in a mug.

Cortisol Regulation

Omega-3 Fatty Acids: Found in fish, flaxseeds, and walnuts, these healthy fats regulate cortisol levels, support brain health, and reduce inflammation—win-win!

Cut Down on Caffeine: I know, I know... caffeine can spike cortisol levels and mess with your hormone balance. Reducing your intake can make a big difference. Your adrenal glands will thank you.

Caffeine and Hormonal imbalances

For those with hormonal imbalance, coffee can be a double-edged sword. Caffeine can potentially exacerbate symptoms by influencing hormone levels and increasing inflammation. Some might not notice any adverse effects, while others might benefit from cutting back.

What You Put In Your Mouth...

Personal Anecdote: As someone who has wrestled with adenomyosis, I noticed significant improvements by moderating my coffee intake. I used to down eight shots of espresso each morning. After taking a nine-month coffee hiatus, I found that one cup a day works wonders for me now. Could coffee be making your adenomyosis worse? Let's delve into the research and my journey to find out.

Swap, Don't Stop: Instead of depriving yourself, crowd out the bad stuff by adding so much good stuff that you naturally have less room for the not-so-great stuff. Think berries, leafy greens, nuts, and seeds. Your brain will thrive on these antioxidants, healthy fats, and vitamins.

Alcohol

Long-term alcohol consumption can affect your body's stress response, potentially increasing cortisol levels and leading to stress-related health issues such as anxiety, depression, and sleep disturbances.
PSA: Alcohol can also increase other various toxins ... such as toxic men, due to temporary impaired judgement.

Impact on the Nervous System: Alcohol impairs the brain regions controlling balance, memory, speech, and judgement, increasing the likelihood of injuries and negative outcomes. Chronic heavy drinking can lead to neuron alterations, reducing their size.

Alcohol's Reach: This small molecule can easily cross membrane barriers, quickly affecting various body parts. It contracts brain tissues, destroys brain cells, and depresses the central nervous system. Over time, excessive drinking can cause serious cognitive and memory issues.

What You Put In Your Mouth...

Understanding how caffeine and alcohol affect your body can help you make more informed choices. Moderation and mindfulness are key, and sometimes a little break can do wonders for your health. Cheers to making choices that make you feel good, inside and out!

Bio-individuality

Let's dive into the fascinating world of bio-individuality—an idea so essential it deserves a spotlight on every wellness stage. Think of the unprocessed app as your backstage pass to the bio-hacker's playground, where one size most certainly does not fit all. Instead, it's your go-to tool for decoding the unique symphony that is your body's nutritional needs.

What exactly is bio-individuality? It's the concept that your body's nutritional and health requirements are as unique as your fingerprint, shaped by a mix of factors even Sherlock Holmes would find intriguing.

1. **Blood Type**: Ever wonder why your friend thrives on steak while you're more of a tofu aficionado? Your blood type might just be the dietary detective behind it.

2. **Genes**: Forget horoscopes—your genetic blueprint influences everything from how you process carbs to why you've got a soft spot for midnight snacks.

3. **Activity Level**: Whether you're a gym regular or more of a Netflix marathoner, your workout habits have a direct line to your metabolism and nutrient needs.

4. **Stress Level**: Chronic stress isn't just a mood killer; it's a metabolic meddler, tweaking hormone levels and messing with digestion in ways that aren't cute.

What You Put In Your Mouth...

5. **Lifestyle**: Your daily routine—even that 3pm caffeine fix—plays a starring role in how your body operates on the inside.

6. **Beliefs**: Whether motivated by culture, personal values, or religious reasons, your dietary choices are part of your bio-individual makeup—be it vegan, keto, or somewhere in between.

7. **Gut Health**: Your microbiome is the unsung hero of your digestive and immune systems. A healthy gut is like having a backstage crew that keeps the whole show running smoothly.

8. **Habits**: From sleep patterns to snack preferences, your long-standing habits are the directors of your body's daily performance.

There's more to it:

- **Age**: Your body's dietary needs evolve over time, proving that ageing changes more than just appearances—it also alters nutritional priorities.
- **Gender**: Men and women have different nutritional requirements—think Mars and Venus on a plate.
- **Health Conditions**: Chronic illnesses, allergies, and intolerances turn your dietary needs into a bespoke menu, tailored just for you.
- **Environment**: Factors like climate and pollution levels invisibly shape your health needs.
- **Access to Food**: The quality and availability of your food can distinguish between thriving and merely surviving.
- **Emotional Health**: Your mental state influences not just your mood but also your eating habits.

- **Sleep**: Quality shut-eye is the unsung hero of metabolism and overall health, akin to a nightly rebooting of your system.

Each of these factors weaves together to form your unique health and nutritional profile, proving that a one-size-fits-all approach to wellness is as effective as a chocolate teapot. Personalised health is not just a luxury—it's a necessity in navigating the intricate tapestry of your bio-individuality.

Nutrients over Calories

The old "calories in, calories out" model has the same vibes as those outdated fashion rules like "no white after Labor Day"—overly simplistic and, frankly, just a bit out of touch. Sure, calories matter, but there's so much more happening beneath the surface, kind of like what's going on behind those Instagram filters. Let's peel back the layers, shall we?

1. **Not All Calories Are Created Equal—Kind of Like Shoes**

Imagine trying to walk a mile in six-inch stilettos versus comfy sneakers. Technically, you're walking the same distance, but one of these options will burn a lot more energy (and possibly your dignity), the same logic applies to food. Sure, a protein-packed grilled chicken breast and a doughnut might have similar calorie counts, but your body is working much harder to break down that chicken. Proteins, carbs, and fats aren't just numbers on a box—they each have different "workout routines" in your body. Some take more effort (hello, protein), while others just waltz right through (looking at you, refined sugar).

What You Put In Your Mouth...

2. **Hormones—The Frenemies of Weight Loss**

Ah, hormones. If calories are the plot of a rom-com, hormones are the unpredictable best friend who throws a spanner in the works. Cortisol, insulin, leptin—all these characters are up to their own tricks. Insulin, for example, is like that friend who tells you to save money but then persuades you to blow it all on a shopping spree. When it's too high, your body just keeps storing fat, no matter how saintly your calorie-counting. Even if you're in a calorie deficit, if your hormones are out of whack, it's equivalent to trying to lose weight while someone keeps secretly ordering takeout to your door.

3. **Gut Feelings (Literally) Matter**

Let's talk about the other gut instinct—your microbiome. Those trillions of little bacteria in your digestive system are basically the hipster baristas of your metabolism. Some are great at turning food into energy, while others hoard it like it's an avocado toast shortage. Depending on the state of your gut health, two people could eat the exact same meal, but one might absorb more calories than the other. Your body's response to calories depends on who's running the café inside your belly.

4. **Metabolic Slowdown—The Energy-Saving Mode of Your Body**

If you've ever had your phone battery die at 20% because it went into some sneaky power-saving mode, you've got a glimpse of what your metabolism does when you consistently eat fewer calories. Your body, ever the survivalist, slows everything down to conserve energy as it's preparing for the next apocalypse (or juice cleanse). Voilà, weight loss screeches to a halt and that kale salad isn't doing its job anymore.

5. **It's About Quality, Not Just Quantity—Kind of Like a Good Friend**
You wouldn't hang out with people who drain your energy, right? (If you do, we will get to you later). The same goes for your nutrition. You can fill your plate with the same number of calories, but a meal of whole foods and nutrient-dense goodies is like hanging out with friends who make you feel alive, versus junk food that's basically the toxic friend group of the food world. Sure, a cupcake might offer the same caloric intake as a handful of nuts, but your body handles them very differently. One leaves you nourished with sustainable brain energy and focus, the other leaves you in a sugar coma.

6. **The Emotional Side—Because We're More Than Just Numbers**
Here's the kicker: food isn't just fuel; it's also a mood lifter, a boredom buster, a stress reliever—you name it. Counting calories might work in a vacuum, but in real life, we've got feelings, stress, and the occasional heartbreak. The "calories in, calories out" model doesn't account for that midnight raid of the freezer when Ben & Jerry's become your temporary therapists. In short, it doesn't account for life.

Neural and Emotional Rewiring.

Neural and Emotional Rewiring

Changing a habit is a little like convincing your brain to take a scenic detour instead of the usual route to your favourite café. Go with me on this—you're cruising down a perfectly paved highway—smooth, predictable, and practically autopilot. This route has been your go-to for years, every twist and turn ingrained in your muscle memory. What happens when you decide to carve out a new path / habit? Suddenly, your perfect highway is a dense, uncharted jungle, and you're armed with little more than a blunt machete and a sprinkle of optimistic determination.

When you embark on changing a behaviour, your brain doesn't just sit idly by. Instead, it orchestrates a physiological symphony, with neurons firing off signals like over-caffeinated messengers. Your synapses are the microscopic gaps between neurons where information is exchanged. You may have heard the phrase, "synapses that fire together, wire together." It's the brain's way of saying that the more you repeat a thought or action, the stronger the connection between the neurons involved. Over time, that once-tangled jungle trail starts to resemble a well-trodden path.

Your old habits are the reliable highway—well-travelled, smooth, and utterly predictable. It's why you can drive to work, plan dinner, and wonder why that guy ghosted you—all without missing a turn. The brain, always the efficiency expert, takes the path of least resistance whenever possible and changing a habit means steering your brain off the highway and into the unknown.

Initially, this new route is fraught with obstacles—vines of self-doubt, swamps of resistance, and maybe even a few metaphorical snakes. Every step demands your full attention, as your brain's prefrontal cortex, the

decision-making HQ, works overtime to clear the way. Meanwhile, the old highway calls out like a siren, promising ease and comfort.
This is why change feels draining—it physically is.
This is why it is vital to be compassionate and gentle with yourself throughout this time of change.

Fortunately, your brain is equipped with neuroplasticity—its built-in GPS that recalculates and learns new routes. With practice, this new path through the jungle becomes more defined. The synapses involved start firing together more frequently, strengthening their connections. Eventually, that once treacherous jungle trail transforms into a smooth road, just as familiar as the old highway.

During this transition, you might feel like an explorer deciphering an ancient map with faded ink. The resistance you encounter isn't failure; it's your brain clinging to the familiar. Each time you choose the new path, you're forging new neural connections. Over time, your brain's reward system kicks in, offering little dopamine boosts, making the new behaviour feel natural.

Soon enough, the new habit becomes second nature. You've reprogrammed your brain, and the new route is now your default. Much like discovering a faster, more scenic route to your favourite café, you'll wonder why you ever stuck to the old highway. Changing a habit requires patience, persistence, and a touch of self-compassion. Remember, each imperfect attempt at the new behaviour strengthens those neural connections.

Neural and Emotional Rewiring

The next time you're struggling to break a habit, think of it as guiding your brain through an exciting new jungle—one that, with time, will lead you to healthier and happier destinations. Before you know it, you'll be navigating with the ease of a seasoned explorer, machete in hand. There are exercises for you to complete at the back of this book to assist with neural rewiring.

Neural and Emotional Rewiring

Your beliefs are like a pair of glasses you never take off. They colour your perception of the world, shaping how you interpret everything you see and experience. For example, if you believe that the world is a dangerous place, you'll spot danger in the most benign situations. You'll see that harmless cloud as a storm brewing, not the fluffy bunny your friend might see. The reality you perceive is largely a reflection of your beliefs based on your past experiences, not an objective truth.

We've all heard the phrase, "Our beliefs shape our reality."
It's practically self-help wallpaper at this point, but have you ever paused to truly grasp what it means?
I always thought I did. I knew that my worldview was coloured by my unique blend of biases, experiences, and quirks. I understood that the people in my life are a reflection of my own conditioning, and if someone didn't particularly like me, it probably had more to do with their background and own biases then with me (not that it didn't still sting).
I understood all of this intellectually. I tried to keep my biases in check, to stay aware of the beliefs I carried around, always asking myself:
Is this belief helping me, or is this belief holding me back?

Here's the kicker: most of our beliefs are buried so deep in the subconscious, we're not even aware that they exist. I realised I was walking around making choices, yet had no idea why I was making them.
It was the equivalent to walking around with spinach in my teeth -
it's impacting my life and how others percieve me, while I am blissfully unaware.

This is where I would like to introduce 'confirmation bias', why our brains are obsessed with being right - even when it can lead to the wrong situation, or wrong relationship.

Neural and Emotional Rewiring

Our brains absolutely love being "right"—it is awarding ourselves a gold star for sticking to the familiar script, even if this script is a toxic relationship. Why? Because predictability feels safe, and safety is our brain's number one priority.

When things align with what we already believe (subconsciously or consciously), our brain relaxes, thinking, "Ah, yes, we know this one, no surprises here." This feeling of certainty even provides our brain a little dopamine boost, our brain's way of patting itself on the back for avoiding the discomfort of questioning what it already "knows."

Confirmation bias feeds off this: we notice evidence that supports our beliefs, happily ignoring or pushing away anything that doesn't fit.

This can be problematic when the comfort of "being right" becomes blinding, especially in the realm of relationships. When certain behaviours or dynamics—even toxic ones—become familiar, our brain starts equating them with safety. It prefers the illusion of stability to the risk of change, no matter how unhealthy the situation.

While we might logically know a relationship isn't good for us, our brain clings to the familiarity, mistaking routine for security and resisting the steps that could lead to something genuinely healthy.

The brain would rather feel "right" in a bad relationship than risk the unknowns of finding a better one.

This is why understanding and being conscious of the beliefs that we hold is extremely powerful, in fact, it creates our entire reality and experience of life. Most of our beliefs, unfortunately, are not conscious, we seemingly drive through life, not knowing who is driving the car, where we are heading or why.

Neural and Emotional Rewiring

Changing your beliefs isn't about pretending everything is perfect. It's about rewiring your brain to see possibilities where you used to see obstacles. This isn't slapping on a smile and ignoring reality; it's about consciously choosing to focus on what's constructive. Think of it as an interior redesign of your mind, swapping out the gloomy, outdated decor for something brighter and more functional.

Thanks to neuroplasticity, your brain is always ready to adapt and with consistent effort you can reprogram your neural pathways, creating new patterns of thought. It's a mental spring cleaning, where you clear out the old, unhelpful clutter and make room for new, empowering beliefs. When you focus on the positive, you're not just boosting your mood; you're changing the way your brain operates. A positive mindset can lead to:

1. **Improved Mental Health:** Less anxiety and depression, more contentment.
2. **Better Decision-Making:** Optimism opens up your ability to think clearly and creatively.
3. **Increased Resilience:** A positive outlook helps you bounce back from setbacks more quickly.

Changing your thoughts isn't just about feeling better; it's about changing your life. When you believe in your ability to succeed, you're more likely to take the actions needed to make success a reality. Your brain, rewired for positivity, starts to spot opportunities where it once saw only problems. This shift in perspective can lead to tangible changes – in your career, your relationships, and your overall well-being.

Neural and Emotional Rewiring

1. **Identify Negative Thoughts:** Start by paying attention to the automatic negative thoughts that pop into your head. I find that writing them down can help me become more aware of patterns and ruminating thoughts which then creates the conscious awareness to actively re-write a new belief.

   I have a notes thread on my phone titled 'brain rewiring' where I write my old thought, then the replacement 'new thought'.

   There is a section at the back of this book for you to begin practising this.

2. **Fact-Check Your Thoughts:** Are these thoughts based on reality, or are they just your brain's old, unhelpful patterns? Challenge them by asking yourself if they're true, if there's another way to look at the situation, or if you're just defaulting to the old habit of seeing the negative.

3. **Practice Gratitude:** It may sound like a cliché, but focusing on what you're grateful for can subtly recalibrate your brain's focus from what's wrong to what's right. Think of it as directing a spotlight toward the brighter aspects of your life, making them more visible and accessible. However, let's not mistake this for toxic positivity or disingenuous gratitude. The notion that "you can't be angry or sad if you're grateful" is something I staunchly disagree with. It's entirely possible to experience conflicting emotions simultaneously—gratitude can coexist with disappointment, sadness, or anger, and all these emotions are equally valid.

   We don't rank emotions as better or worse; while some may be more pleasant to experience, each one serves a purpose. Practising gratitude isn't about ignoring the unpleasant; it's about acknowledging that our brains are hardwired for survival. Left on autopilot, we're inclined to dwell on perceived threats, whether it's a tense email from your boss or the unanswered text from that guy who ghosted you. Our default setting is to fixate on the negative because we crave resolution to stay safe. Cultivating an active focus on gratitude is about gradually reprogramming that autopilot response—creating a more balanced outlook between fear and excitement for life.

4. **Surround Yourself with Positivity:** The people you spend time with can influence your mindset. Surround yourself with those who uplift you and encourage you to see the good in situations.

Focusing on the positive doesn't mean ignoring reality or sugar-coating life. It's about training your brain to see the full picture – both the challenges and the opportunities. By actively working to change your thoughts, you're setting yourself up for a more successful, fulfilling life. Swap those doom-and-gloom glasses for a pair that highlights possibilities, and watch how your world begins to transform.

Neuroplasticity.

(expanded)

Neuroplasticity

Let's expand on the fabulous world of neuroplasticity, the brain's equivalent of a glow-up, but way more impressive than a simple makeover. Think of your brain as the ultimate, top-tier GPS—sure, it can guide you down the usual routes you've taken for years, but with a little effort, it can also reroute, rebuild, and even create entirely new roads that lead to much better destinations. This magic trick is called neuroplasticity, and it's your brain's ability to reorganize, adapt, and even recover from some pretty major blows—we're talking trauma, injury, or just the wear and tear of everyday life.

Imagine your brain not as something fixed or set in stone (thankfully!), but more like a moldable clay. It's not plastic, of course—there's no Tupperware up there—but it is flexible. Neuroplasticity is all about how your brain can change its structure and functions in response to what you're doing, thinking, and experiencing. Whether you're learning a new language or trying to recover after a traumatic brain injury, your brain is constantly updating its software, creating new pathways or reinforcing old ones.

Neuroplasticity

There are two main types of neuroplasticity:

Functional Plasticity: This is when your brain relocates a job from one part to another. Think of it like when your favorite café closes, and you find another one that still serves great coffee. After a stroke or injury, for example, the brain can move certain functions from the damaged area to a healthy one. Hello, adaptability!

Structural Plasticity: This is your brain's ability to physically change its structure because of learning or experience. It's like redecorating your house—except instead of new curtains, your brain is busy growing neurons and making connections. It's the reason learning new skills actually reshapes the brain.

Like a top-tier personal trainer, neuroplasticity helps your brain stay fit, nimble, and ready for anything. It's the gift that keeps on giving.
When your brain is flexible, here's what happens:

You'll strengthen existing skills and boost your cognitive abilities.
Recovery from things like strokes or brain injuries becomes possible because the brain can rewire and take on new roles.
It can help reverse declines in function or adapt to aging, ensuring your brain stays sharp. So yes, neuroplasticity is basically your brain's version of staying forever young.

In the past, scientists believed that once you hit adulthood, your brain was as malleable as a brick wall. Thankfully, we've learned the brain continues to evolve throughout life. Whether you're 25 or 85, your brain is always in the process of remodeling itself—like an HGTV show on loop. Neuroplasticity isn't just for recovery either. When you challenge your brain, through learning or new experiences, it adapts. Want to speak Italian? Neuroplasticity has you covered. Pick up rock climbing? Your brain is already figuring out how to keep you from falling off that cliff.

How do you get in on this brain-boosting action?
It's all about creating the right environment and habits to support neuroplasticity. **Here's how:**

Learn a new skill: We are talking piano or painting.
Travel somewhere new.
Dive into books, create art, or try your hand at writing.
Your brain thrives in environments where it's being pushed in new ways.

Get Plenty of Sleep: While you're snoozing, your brain is busy growing and repairing dendrites (those little connectors between neurons). So that extra hour of sleep might be doing more for your cognitive abilities than you think. Set up a good sleep routine—your brain will thank you in ways you won't even realize, from better memory to quicker learning.

Exercise Regularly: Yes, sweating it out doesn't just make your body feel good—it's like a personal training session for your brain. Regular physical activity boosts neuroplasticity by increasing the production of brain-derived neurotrophic factor (BDNF), a protein that promotes the growth of new neurons. Think of BDNF as your brain's secret sauce for staying sharp. Aim for at least 150 minutes of moderate exercise a week. Walking, swimming, dancing—it all counts. Your brain doesn't care about fancy routines, just that you're moving.

Neuroplasticity

Practice Mindfulness: Mindfulness isn't just for zen moments—it's also a superpower for your brain's plasticity. By staying present and focused, you help your brain strengthen its neural networks. Think of mindfulness as upgrading your brain's operating system—it clears out the junk files and makes room for better functionality.

Play More Games: Brain games aren't just for kids. Engaging in strategic games such as puzzles, board games, or even video games can enhance your brain's ability to rewire itself. Play is serious business for neuroplasticity.

Neuroplasticity is the ultimate self-care for your brain. It's never too late to start giving your mind the environment it needs to grow and adapt. Whether you're learning a new hobby, playing games, or just getting enough sleep, you're setting your brain up for its best life.

The Reward / Effort Ratio.

The Reward / Effort Ratio

Ah, the noble pursuit of self-improvement – often derailed by our own love of comfort. You set out to become a morning jogger, picturing yourself gracefully gliding through the park at dawn. While in reality, you end up scrolling through social media, double-tapping on other people's fitness posts instead. Enter the reward/effort ratio, your new best friend in the quest for change. The trick is to make the effort so minimal and the reward so appealing that you can't help but succeed.

Ever told yourself, "I'll start tomorrow," only to find that tomorrow-you is just as unmotivated as today-you? This is because nothing changes between today and tomorrow, so don't expect a sudden burst of enthusiasm. Your brain, ever the creature of habit, will cling to the familiar. It's like trying to convince yourself to take a detour through that jungle we mentioned earlier, when your brain is perfectly content cruising down the smooth, well-paved highway of old habits.

To outsmart your brain's resistance, start with micro changes – tiny, manageable adjustments that seem almost too easy to bother with. It's like sneaking veggies into a child's dinner: subtle, small, and surprisingly effective.

1. **1 minute:** This is the warm up, zero room for resistance.
2. **5 minutes:** Just five minutes. It's so little time that it barely feels like a commitment.
3. **10 minutes:** Double the time, but still within the realm of "I can totally do this."
4. **15 minutes**: Now you're starting to make actual progress, and your brain is beginning to adjust to the new routine.

The Reward / Effort Ratio

The smaller the change, the less resistance you'll encounter. It's like coaxing your brain out of its comfort zone with baby steps rather than dragging it kicking and screaming into a new habit.

Remember, your brain is wired to do what it knows. It's built for survival, which means sticking with the familiar, even if the familiar is binge-watching Netflix instead of going for a run. By making micro changes, you're gently guiding your brain into accepting new behaviours, driving along the highway with a short off road detour rather than signing up for a week long hike through a jungle.

Here's the key to making these new habits stick: the reward. Your brain needs to believe that the reward for your new habit far outweighs the effort required. If the effort is minimal, and the reward is enticing, you're more likely to stick with it. It's basic psychology – even your dog understands it. Give a dog a treat for a trick, and they'll be doing backflips for you in no time.

When it comes to making changes, you need to stack the deck in your favour. Make the effort as small as possible, the reward as enticing as possible, and your brain will be more likely to cooperate. Over time, those micro changes add up, and before you know it, you're not just a jogger, you're a marathon runner. Start small, reward yourself often, and watch as your brain rewires itself for success.

And please, remember to be gentle with yourself and support yourself in this wild time of transition. Change, no matter how small, can feel like an existential threat to your brain. It's as though deciding to switch from lounging on the couch to taking a brisk walk sets off alarms, with your mind acting as if you're facing down a sabre-toothed tiger. The familiar neural pathways your brain clings to are cosy, predictable, and—let's be honest—sometimes a little too comfortable, even when they no longer serve you. When you step into the unknown, even for something positive, your brain and body can revolt, triggering full-blown physiological panic, as if you're diving headfirst into chaos.

This is where working with a trauma-informed practitioner can make all the difference. These professionals are skilled in teaching your nervous system to adapt to change in a way that doesn't send you spiralling into fight-or-flight mode. By implementing strategies like breathwork, somatic exercises, or mindful movement, they help rewire the body's stress responses. Instead of letting change barrel through your defences, you'll gradually learn how to embrace it, working with your nervous system rather than against it. Over time, these calming techniques train your body to handle shifts with grace, allowing you to make healthier choices without feeling like you're teetering on the edge of disaster.

I would be so honoured to assist you with this transformation, head to unprocessedapp.com to book in a session with a trauma informed practitioner today!

CREATING YOUR OWN SAFE

SPACE.

Creating Your Own Safe Space

Alright, let's have a heart-to-heart about nourishment. When we talk about nourishing our bodies, it's not just about what's on your plate or in your glass. Catching up with a dear friend? That's nourishment. Strolling through nature? Pure nourishment. Soaking up some sunshine before diving into screen time? Yup, nourishment. Putting your phone away an hour before bed? You guessed it, nourishment.

These lifestyle choices are just as, if not more crucial than the vitamins and minerals in your meals. They send signals to your body that play a big role in how it develops and responds. Think of them as the star roles of your nourishment, and the nutrients that you consume as the supporting cast.

You can chug green juice like it's going out of fashion and run like you're training for a marathon, but if you're living in a constant state of fight-or-flight (hello, red zone), your body is too busy prepping for an imaginary tiger chase to focus on digesting food properly. All those carefully chosen nutrients? They're just passing through without stopping to chat. Sometimes, stressing over having a perfect diet can do more harm than if you just relaxed and enjoyed a slice of pizza.
Seriously, chill and let the pepperoni do its thing.

Feeling overwhelmed and a bit down while trying super hard to be upbeat? Exhausted but can't seem to switch off? Struggling to step away from being 'productive'? These are red flags that you're camped out in the Sympathetic Nervous System—the fight-or-flight zone.
Running on adrenaline, caffeine, and muscle glycogen instead of the slow, sustainable energy from stored fats... ever wonder why your 16 cardio sessions a week aren't getting you results? Well, now you know.

Creating Your Own Safe Space

Nourishing your body goes beyond food and drink. It's about creating a life that supports your overall well-being.

When I dived into the world of integrative nutrition, I was blown away by the power of the nervous system. Picture this: studying over 100 different diets and seeing how they affected different people. It became clear that living a long, healthy, and happy life isn't just about what you eat or drink, the secret sauce lies in these five pillars that keep our nervous system in check, which then keeps our hormones happy.

1. **Stress**: Safety, Sleep, Sex and Sense of Self
2. **Purpose**: Presence and Perspective
3. **Attention**: Acceptance, Awareness and Attention
4. **Community**: Communication and Connection
5. **Environment**: Energy and Exercise

Stress.

Stress

Welcome to the rollercoaster of the 21st century—where hustle culture reigns supreme and the pressure to be perpetually productive has us all strapped in tight. From dawn to dusk, we're juggling meetings, deadlines, and to-do lists that never seem to shorten. In the quest to achieve more, we've transformed rest into a luxury rather than a necessity, leaving us running on fumes rather than fuel.

In this chapter, we'll delve into the pervasive impact of stress on our bodies and minds. We'll explore how trauma embeds itself deep within us, manifesting in ways we might not even recognise. It's time to break the cycle, to understand that perfection is an illusion, and that managing stress is about more than just checking items off a list. It's about finding peace amidst the chaos, and learning to be kind to ourselves in the process.

It seems as though stress has become a constant companion. It's a sneaky adversary, weaving its way into every aspect of our lives. For me, it's been a relentless battle with my own body, contending with hormonal imbalances and the chronic pain of adenomyosis. Each day is a balancing act, trying to manage physical discomfort while keeping up with the demands of a fast-paced life.

Let's not forget the emotional toll. Life throws curveballs when we least expect them—breakups, career setbacks, and the constant comparison game we play on social media. The irony of modern life is that we're stressed about reducing stress. We're bombarded with advice on how to eat perfectly, exercise daily, meditate, and somehow fit in self-care, all while maintaining a smile on our face and a calm demeanour.

Stress

It's exhausting. The pressure to do everything "right" can be overwhelming, creating a paradox where the pursuit of a stress-free life becomes a major source of stress itself. We strive to balance our nutrition, our schedules, and our minds, yet often find ourselves falling short, caught in a cycle of guilt and frustration. We don't just judge ourselves for how we use our time, but we judge ourselves for how we feel - accepting happiness and declining all other emotions, because what use could they possibly have in our lives anyway?

This apprehension and avoidance of any emotion that is not 'happy' or 'inspired' creates a dissociation with self, trying to push away the emotion that we judge as negative, rather than inviting them in like an old friend that is here to let us know that something is up and action is required. Feeling is healing and sometimes, all that is required is for us to sit with this discomfort to let it do its thing and complete its necessary process within the body. The key is feeling it, without having to act through it - we will talk more on this later.

Whether it's work deadlines, family responsibilities, or global events, stressors can pile up, taking a toll on our physical and mental health. But what exactly happens when we experience stress, and how does our body respond?

As we touched on before, when faced with a stressful situation, our body's ancient survival mechanism kicks in: the fight-or-flight response. This involves the release of stress hormones such as cortisol and adrenaline, which prepare the body to either confront or flee from the perceived threat. Heart rate increases, muscles tense, and breathing becomes rapid. While this response can be lifesaving in acute situations, chronic activation can lead to a host of health issues.

Stress

- **Cardiovascular System**: Persistent stress can contribute to hypertension, increased risk of heart attacks, and stroke. The continuous strain on the heart and blood vessels can have long-lasting consequences.
- **Immune System**: Chronic stress suppresses the immune system, making the body more susceptible to infections and slowing down the healing process.
- **Digestive System**: Stress doesn't just mess with your mind; it throws your gut into chaos too, often leading to conditions like irritable bowel syndrome (IBS), acid reflux, or even ulcers.
  Stress levels matter more than what you eat.
  Why? Because stress doesn't just influence digestion—it dictates your cravings, your willpower, your mindfulness, your motivation, and your overall attitude. At a deeper level, as we've already explored, stress can directly impact your body's ability to properly digest and absorb nutrients. In short, you could be eating all the kale in the world, but if stress has the wheel, it's like trying to fuel a car with a clogged engine.
- **Musculoskeletal System**: Muscle tension, a common stress response, can cause headaches, back pain, and general discomfort.
- **Endocrine System**: Long-term stress disrupts the hormonal balance, contributing to conditions such as diabetes and thyroid disorders.

Trauma, whether from a single event or prolonged exposure to distressing situations, leaves an indelible mark on the body and mind. Our bodies can store these traumatic experiences in ways that subtly but significantly influence our daily lives.

Stress

The concept of somatic memory suggests that trauma can be stored in the body. This means that even if we consciously forget a traumatic event, our bodies may retain a physical memory of it.
This can manifest in various ways:

- **Chronic Pain**: Unresolved trauma can lead to chronic pain conditions, such as fibromyalgia, where the pain is widespread and persistent without a clear physical cause.

- **Muscle Tension**: Certain muscles may remain in a state of tension, guarding against perceived threats, which can result in pain and discomfort.

- **Posture and Movement**: Trauma can alter the way we hold ourselves and move. For instance, someone who has experienced abuse might unconsciously hunch their shoulders as if to protect themselves.

Trauma doesn't just affect us physically; it also shapes our behaviours and interactions, often in ways we aren't fully aware of.Trauma can make us more susceptible to emotional triggers; situations that remind us of the original trauma, even in subtle ways, can provoke strong emotional reactions. This can include:

- **Anxiety and Panic Attacks**: Certain sights, sounds, or even smells can trigger anxiety or panic, seemingly out of nowhere.

- **Avoidance Behaviour**: We might find ourselves avoiding places, people, or activities that remind us of the traumatic event, limiting our experiences and interactions.

Stress

Trauma can influence the way we relate to others, often leading to patterns that reflect our internal struggles:

- **Trust Issues**: Trauma, especially from abuse or betrayal, can make it difficult to trust others. This can lead to difficulties in forming and maintaining relationships.
- **Attachment Styles**: Our early experiences of trauma can shape our attachment styles, making us overly dependent, distant, or fearful in relationships.

To manage the pain of trauma, we often develop coping mechanisms, some of which can be maladaptive:

- **Substance Use**: Turning to alcohol, drugs, or other substances to numb emotional pain is a common but harmful coping strategy.
- **Disassociation**: In response to overwhelming stress or trauma, some individuals may disconnect from reality, experiencing periods of disassociation where they feel detached from their body or surroundings.

Another strategy is minimisation of the trauma. It might feel like a good way to cope with the pain, to decrease how bad it hurts in our mind and sometimes this is necessary but it is not a long term solution. Dealing is not the same thing as healing; dealing allows you to cope until you are strong and stable enough to put in the hard yards of healing. Minimising trauma is like trying to put a Band-Aid on a broken bone—it might cover up the surface, but it doesn't fix the real damage underneath. People often minimise their trauma as a coping mechanism, convincing themselves that "it wasn't that bad" or "others have it worse." While this might provide temporary relief, it's ultimately a way of avoiding the deep work needed to heal. Imagine trying to ignore a fire alarm by telling yourself it's just a distant car horn—sooner or later, that fire is going to demand your attention.

When we downplay our experiences, we're essentially telling ourselves that our pain isn't valid, which only compounds the problem. It's like trying to carry a heavy suitcase up a flight of stairs while pretending it's as light as a feather—eventually, your arms are going to give out. Minimisation can lead to unresolved issues festering beneath the surface, manifesting in physical symptoms, anxiety, or even explosive emotional reactions at seemingly minor triggers.

The tricky part about minimisation is that it often sneaks in under the guise of being "strong" or "resilient." Society sometimes praises people for "getting over it" quickly, but real strength lies in acknowledging the full weight of our experiences and choosing to heal anyway.
How do we break free from the minimisation trap? Start by giving yourself permission to feel the full scope of your emotions—no matter how "small" or "insignificant" they might seem in comparison to someone else's. Trauma isn't a competition, and pain is pain. Just like you wouldn't compare a sprained ankle to a broken leg, you shouldn't compare your trauma to anyone else's. Healing begins when we stop minimising and start validating our own experiences, no matter how uncomfortable that might be.

In short, while minimising might seem like a handy shortcut through the rough patches, it's more like a detour that leads you back to the same unresolved pain, just with more baggage in tow. Real healing requires us to drop the act and confront our trauma head-on—acknowledging that even the smallest cuts deserve care.

Stress

Understanding the profound impact of stress and trauma on our bodies and minds is the first step towards healing.

Various therapeutic approaches can help:

- **Psychotherapy**: Techniques such as Cognitive Behavioural Therapy (CBT) and Eye Movement Desensitisation and Reprocessing (EMDR) can help process and integrate traumatic memories.
- **Body-Oriented Therapies**: Approaches like somatic experiencing and trauma-sensitive yoga focus on releasing trauma stored in the body.
- **Mindfulness and Relaxation Techniques**: Practices such as meditation, deep breathing, and progressive muscle relaxation can help calm the nervous system and reduce stress.

Stress and trauma are pervasive elements of the human experience, leaving marks that go far beyond the immediate moments of crisis. By understanding how these forces shape our bodies and minds, we can begin to unravel their hold on us, paving the way for healing and resilience. Remember, seeking help and acknowledging these challenges is a powerful step towards reclaiming control and fostering a healthier, more balanced life.

Stress: Safety

Creating a safe environment—both internally and externally—is fundamental to achieving a healthy and fulfilling life, especially for those recovering from trauma. Establishing safety involves multiple facets of our lives, each playing a critical role in our overall well-being.

1. Working Within Your Own Boundaries: You don't need permission to set boundaries, but let me give it to you anyway: Your peace matters. Your needs matter. And if you keep living as if they don't, you'll pay for it—with your energy, your happiness, and eventually, your health.

Let me ask you this: how often do you agree to things that drain you, just to avoid the discomfort of saying no? How many times have you felt resentful because you gave more than you had to give? Here's the hard truth: every time you abandon yourself to please someone else, you're teaching the world that your limits don't matter. And if you don't respect your boundaries, no one else will either.

Boundaries aren't walls to keep people out; they're doors that let the right energy in. They're not just about saying no—they're about saying yes to yourself. To your mental clarity. To your physical health. To your right to feel safe, respected, and whole. Without them, you're running on empty, pouring from a cup that's bone-dry, while quietly wondering why everything feels so damn hard.

This isn't just about self-care; it's survival. The most loving act you can ever do—for yourself and everyone around you—is to honour your limits. Start asking: Am I doing this for them, or am I doing it for me? Start choosing yourself unapologetically, because when you do, your life will change. By choosing yourself unapologetically, you are also giving the people in your life permission to do the same, imagine that, a whole world where we all take responsibility for our own wellbeing.

Stress: Safety

Boundaries aren't selfish. They're necessary. Without them, you'll burn out, break down, and resent the people you're bending over backwards to accommodate. With them, you create space for what truly matters—for the relationships, opportunities, and experiences that nourish you instead of depleting you. This is your permission to choose yourself. To draw the line. To stop apologising for taking up space in your own life. Your future self will thank you. And if anyone is upset by your boundaries? That's their problem to solve—not yours. *Big sigh of relief*

2. Having a resource: Eventually, you will develop the skills and strategies to become your own resource and know that no matter what happens, who stays, who goes, and what life throws at you - you will be ok. In the meantime and especially in the early stages of this journey, I suggest working with a trauma informed practitioner who is specifically trained to understand the impact of your trauma, how to navigate it and how to support you effectively without causing further harm.

Think about it as driving to a new destination for the first time, you wouldn't expect yourself to magically guess how to get there without a GPS - in life, healing the trauma is the new destination and your trauma informed practitioner is the GPS. Eventually, you can turn the GPS off and navigate yourself, but if you are as geographically challenged as I am, it might take a few trips to the destination before you are ready for that, and sometimes you might want to pop the GPS on, just in case.

3. Decreasing substances that can impact your long term mood and healing such as coffee and alcohol: Reducing stimulants and depressants can help stabilise mood and improve overall health, creating a safer internal environment. We spoke about this.

Stress: Safety

4. **Mindful Relationships:** During this phase of healing, it's essential to be acutely aware of the energy you invite into your life. Healing is an incredibly demanding process—a true hero's journey. It takes immense courage to face the fears that have been tucked away and allow yourself to fully experience uncomfortable emotions, rather than escaping from them. It's no wonder that people often turn to distractions like a pill or a drink; feeling the pain head-on is hard work.

You deserve—and need—love, compassion, and understanding, both from yourself and from those around you. At this point in your life (and honestly, always), it's vital to be relentless yet gentle in distancing yourself from relationships that disrupt your peace, especially as you tread through this new and challenging terrain.

People often serve as mirrors, reflecting the aspects of ourselves that require deeper investigation. When someone triggers discomfort within you, it's a signal that there's something within yourself that might need attention. This isn't to suggest that you avoid these triggers—on the contrary, they're crucial for growth. However, you have full permission to lovingly distance yourself from those who are judgmental, negative, or simply drain your energy, particularly when so much of it is being devoted to your own healing.
Surround yourself with relationships that are nurturinq and supportive, those that provide the emotional safety you need to continue on this path of recovery.

5. **Fulfilling Work:** Engaging in work that brings you fulfillment contributes to a sense of purpose and stability.

Stress: Safety

Types of Safety

- **Physical Safety:** Ensuring your environment is free from harm.
- **Emotional Safety:** Feeling secure in expressing your emotions without fear of judgement.
- **Financial Safety:** Having financial stability and security.
- **Institutional Safety:** Trust in the systems and institutions you interact with.
- **Relational Safety:** Feeling safe in your relationships.
- **Societal Safety:** Living in a society that respects your rights and dignity.
- **Spiritual Safety:** Feeling secure in your spiritual or religious practices.

Judith Lewis Herman, in her book "Trauma and Recovery," emphasises the importance of establishing safety as the first stage of trauma recovery. She states, "The first, and perhaps most important, stage of trauma recovery is about establishing safety. People affected by trauma tend to feel unsafe in their bodies and in their relationships with others. This stage might last weeks, months, or even years, depending on the level of trauma. Everyone's journey and timeline is different."
This stage focuses on developing self-soothing and self-care skills to increase emotional and behavioural stabilisation, helping manage urges to abuse substances, alcohol, and self-harm.

Establishing safety can mean the difference between a therapeutic release and re-traumatisation during the healing process.

Stress: Safety

Re-traumatisation occurs when a person re-experiences a previously traumatic event, consciously or unconsciously. This can be triggered by various stressors that mimic the original trauma environment, such as smells, physical spaces, or even new relationships.

Symptoms of Trauma or Re-traumatisation:

- Flashbacks and nightmares
- Anxiety or fear
- Difficulty concentrating
- Trouble sleeping
- Fatigue
- Social isolation and avoidance
- Intense negative emotions
- Inability to control emotions
- Strong physical reactions to triggers

Re-traumatisation can manifest differently for each individual. For some, it can cause physical shutdown and dissociation, reflecting the initial trauma response.

Understanding the triggers and symptoms of re-traumatisation can help manage and prevent it. Triggers can include:

- Evaluations from clinicians
- Interviews with reporters
- Conversations with friends and family
- Disrespect of emotional boundaries
- Situations involving undressing or physical restraints
- Anniversaries of traumatic events
- Media depictions of similar trauma

Holistic Assessment for Overall Well-being

- **Personal:** Individual life recollections
- **Physiological:** Biological and physical needs
- **Sociological:** Family history and demographics
- **Psychological:** Mental health and emotional well-being
- **Cultural:** Values and customs
- **Spiritual:** Religious practices and values
- **Legal:** Criminal and civil history

Safety is the foundation of trauma recovery. By addressing and securing different areas of safety in our lives, we pave the way for genuine healing and personal growth. Understanding and managing re-traumatisation is crucial to ensure a supportive and nurturing environment for recovery.

If you have experienced sexual assault, domestic violence, or another form of trauma, you are not alone and immediate help is available.

1800 Respect (Call 1800 737 732 or Text 0458 737 732) is a national domestic and sexual violence counselling service available 24 / 7.

Our national suicide helpline service Lifeline is available 24 / 7.
If you need help, please call 13 11 14 or text 0477 13 11 14

Stress: Sleep

Life today can often feel as though you're strapped into the driver's seat of a turbocharged car, careening through deadlines and distractions with barely a second to hit the brakes.
Achieving a good night's sleep? It's less like finding a unicorn and more like spotting a unicorn juggling gymnastic rings while sprinkling glitter—impressive, elusive, and borderline mythical.

Here's the reality check: sleep isn't just a luxury or a cute add-on to your wellness routine. A restorative night of sleep is your body's reset button, the difference between waking up ready to tackle life like Sara Blakely pitching Spanx or trudging through your day feeling like a coffee-fuelled sloth that got side-swiped by reality.

Good sleep isn't just about logging eight hours. It's about quality, consistency, and timing. Dr. Maiken Nedergaard from the University of Rochester describes sleep as the brain's maintenance shift. While you dream, your brain detoxifies, clearing out proteins linked to Alzheimer's and resetting itself for creativity, learning, and memory. Without this process, your brain is a cluttered desk—overwhelmed and inefficient.
Dr. Kenneth Wright Jr. adds that sleep isn't just brain care—it's a full-body repair system. During sleep, everything from blood vessels to your immune system gets its tune-up. Skimp on sleep, and you're cutting these vital processes short, leaving your body vulnerable to disease and dysfunction. Here's the catch: more sleep isn't always better. Oversleeping can signal underlying issues such as sleep disorders, stress, or hormonal imbalances. And no, catching up on the weekend doesn't erase the effects of consistent sleep deprivation.

Stress: Sleep

Why do you suddenly want to text your ex at night? Let's talk about that moment when the clock strikes midnight, and you suddenly feel the overwhelming urge to reconnect with that person. You know the one. During the day, you're composed, confident, and clear-headed. But at night, you're suddenly spiralling, drafting texts, doom-scrolling Instagram, or planning ill-advised heart-to-hearts.

What's happening here? Blame serotonin and melatonin—your brain's chemical see-saw. Serotonin, the "happy hormone," peaks during the day, keeping you upbeat and socially engaged. It's produced in your gut (95% of it, in fact) and the brainstem, with sunlight giving it a boost. As night falls, melatonin takes over, preparing your body for sleep while serotonin dips.

Melatonin is your body's gentle nudge toward bedtime, regulating your sleep-wake cycle. The trade-off is that as serotonin wanes, so does your mood stability. This dip can leave you craving connection—or, more accurately, a quick serotonin hit. Cue the illogical, emotionally driven urge to text your ex or rehash old wounds.

Recognising this seesaw effect helps you pause before hitting "send." Instead of feeding the impulse, try dimming the lights, lighting a candle, or practising deep breathing to settle your body for sleep.

You'll thank yourself in the morning.

If you really need a serotonin hit, have a warm cacao or restorative herbal tea with some honey instead... at least it won't break your heart or dishonour your boundaries my babe... and Yums.

Stress: Sleep

Sleep Saboteurs: What's Getting in the Way?

- **Irregular schedules:** A chaotic routine throws off your body's internal clock.
- **Screen time:** Blue light suppresses melatonin, delaying sleep.
- **Room conditions:** Temperature, darkness, and airflow all impact quality.
- **Stress and safety:** Emotional turmoil or feeling unsafe can keep your nervous system on high alert.
- **Nutrition and substances:** Caffeine, alcohol, and late-night snacks wreak havoc on your sleep cycle.

Understanding your personal sleep patterns is key. How long does it take you to fall asleep? Do you wake up often? Are you groggy or napping during the day? A sleep diary can uncover triggers and patterns, while tools like the Pittsburgh Quality Sleep Index (PSQI) or a sleep study can detect deeper issues.

Practical Tips for Better Sleep

... I could write 5 - 10 dot points here, but the truth is, you know what to do, it's just about actually prioritising yourself enough to do it.
Light a candle, decrease blue light, let yourself unwind and rest.

Sleep affects everything: mood, focus, physical health, and even how you connect with others. Treating it as optional is the same as fuelling a high-performance car with soda—it's not going to end well. Prioritising sleep is the ultimate act of self-care, giving your mind and body the restoration they deserve. Because at the end of the day (pun intended), sleep isn't just about waking up refreshed—it's about living a life that feels full, vibrant, and unshakeable.
And really, isn't that worth putting your phone down for?

Stress: Sleep

Honestly, the best sleep advice that I can give is to actively take steps towards living a life that feels in alignment. Clean your home, clean your energy, live with integrity, make decisions you are proud of, spend time with people that value you, communicate with intention, avoid drama and gossip. Spend time in nature, decrease time online. Breathe deeply, speak kindly to yourself, move your body. Set boundaries, enforce those boundaries, vibe alone until you're valued.

Really fun, completely not clinical advice... if you are really struggling to sleep, try lying on the cold tiles of your kitchen or bathroom floor.

I am pretty sure I heard this strategy in a Taylor Tomlinson stand up comedy special, but I genuinely feel like it is worth a shot.

Stress: Sex (A personal note)

Firstly, a personal note -

To any sexual assault survivors reading this: I see you, and I want you to know that you're not alone. Sex after trauma can be one of the most confusing, emotionally fraught experiences to navigate.
It's a tangled web of feelings—confusion, shame, fear, guilt—and however you feel, you are not alone.

I experienced my first sexual trauma at 14 years old. That experience sent me on a bewildering journey of trying to understand, feel, and experience sex in a way that made sense to me, but nothing did.
I was confused about whether I wanted sex, confused when I didn't, and haunted by a lingering sense that I would never have a "normal" experience of intimacy again.

After that trauma at age 14, I decided that sex shouldn't mean anything to me. I surrendered any sense of control, believing that men would take what they wanted anyway, so why fight it? That belief led me down a painful road of saying "yes" when I didn't mean it—until, at 19, I finally found the strength and wisdom to say "no."

At 21, another sexual trauma by a different person reintroduced that sense of helplessness. After this trauma, I started experiencing panic attacks during sex. The confusion only deepened. I didn't want to talk about the assault—especially not with someone I'd just started dating—but I felt an obligation to warn them: "To no fault of your own, I might have a panic attack during sex. It's not you; it's me. Totally fine—just need to pause, breathe, and then we're good to go."

Stress: Sex (A personal note)

The dread I felt around those conversations was overwhelming. My biggest fear was that my trauma would scare someone off, dampening any potential for romance. It felt deeply unfair—these men hurt me, and yet I'm the one left to carry the weight and navigate its consequences for the rest of my life. I wanted more than anything to just feel 'normal' again. To decide whether or not I would sleep with someone on my own accord, not my traumas.

Even when I found joy in intimacy with someone that I cared for, guilt would creep in. It felt as though I was betraying the younger version of myself who had endured so much pain. How could I allow myself to enjoy something that had also caused so much harm?

Earlier this year, I decided I'd had enough. No more panic attacks.
No more letting trauma define my experiences.
No more carrying this burden. Enough was enough.
Healing looks different for everyone, for me, self-defence training became a game-changer. With a trusted instructor, I worked to desensitise my physical triggers through repeated practice. Learning how to defend myself if someone grabbed me again gave me a newfound sense of safety and confidence. That physical empowerment created a foundation for emotional safety.
Self-defence, working with a trauma informed practitioner, and EFT tapping became the three cornerstones of my healing journey.

One of the most unexpected and transformative steps in my healing was sitting down for coffee with one of the men who assaulted me. I want to be clear: this isn't the right choice for everyone. It requires an immense amount of emotional and physical safety, and in many cases, it may not be appropriate or helpful. But for me, it was a pivotal moment.

Stress: Sex (A personal note)

I had spent 25 years muting myself—avoiding conflict, trying to keep the peace, and valuing others' opinions over my own. That conversation wasn't just about addressing the trauma; it was about reclaiming my voice and stepping into a life where I take responsibility for my own well-being. Healing isn't linear, and triggers still show up. Certain movies, books, situations or even conversations about trauma can affect me, and I've learned to honour my limits. If something feels too overwhelming, I step away—and that's ok.

My panic attacks have largely subsided, and my relationship with sex feels healthier now. Still, I only engage in a sexual relationship with someone I trust enough to share my story with, if needed or wanted. Unexpected triggers can arise, but my safety—physical, emotional, and mental—always comes first.

Healing is hard, messy, and deeply personal. Your wellbeing and ability to feel at peace is worth the effort, and no one has the right to dictate your journey except you.
Always trust your intuition and never let anyone override it.

Stress: Sex

Sex is a natural desire, and it's something that should be celebrated and expressed in a safe, healthy way. It's a beautiful means to deepen a connection with someone who truly deserves your trust and affection. Opening up about sex can sometimes feel uncomfortable or taboo, but these conversations are incredibly important. When we talk openly about sex, we help remove the stigma, leading to healthier and more respectful communication. Now that's something everyone can benefit from.

Unfortunately, the current statistics show us just how crucial it is to prioritise safety and set clear boundaries. In 2024, a study of 5,000 Australians aged 18 to 45 revealed that over 20% had committed an act of sexual violence, ranging from harassment to sharing intimate images and sexual assault. The Australian Bureau of Statistics reported that in 2023, there were 36,318 survivors of sexual assault, with an 11% increase from the previous year. Most of these assaults occurred in residential locations, and nearly 40% were related to family and domestic violence - these statistics only show evidence of the cases that have been reported, unfortunately with the shame and guilt that is all too often associated with violence and abuse, along with the daunting protocols of making a formal report, many incidents go unreported.

It is very important to note that although both women and men are victims of sexual violence and both equally deserve to experience sex in a safe and healthy environment, the current statistics show that 84% of victims are female, and the most common age group is between 10 and 17 years old. Again, these statistics are based on the reported incidents and may not show an honest reflection. One thing that the statistics do highlight is the integral importance of women's safety and the necessity of knowing that you can say "no" at any time. Unfortunately, this is not always an option and it is crucial to understand that if this happens, it is not your fault, and that there is help available.

'Setting boundaries' has become a popular topic of conversation across social platforms. I think that it is important to discuss the very real fear and anxiety that can come up when setting boundaries. This is particularly evident in people who have experienced some form of trauma (which is everyone to a varying degree) and feel a disproportionate emotional response to needing to set a boundary. It can feel genuinely debilitating, perhaps even life threatening because there is a deeper wound that has not been properly addressed and healed yet.

Just like learning to swim or ride a bike, setting boundaries will become easier with experience and practice. It might feel daunting at first, but once you get the hang of it, it becomes second nature. You may fear setting boundaries because you worry about rejection, conflict, being perceived as selfish, or feel a genuine concern for your safety, I know that I do. Here's the thing: boundaries are not barriers, they're more like the gentle fences around a garden that protect your space, energy, and well-being... that sounds lovely doesn't it? Here are some tips:

1. Understand Your Fear

First, it's crucial to identify why you're afraid to set boundaries. Where is this coming from? Is it fear of confrontation? Worry about being disliked? Concern about hurting someone else's feelings? Understanding the root cause of your fear can help you address it more effectively. Once you identify that this fear is coming from a certain (probably childhood) moment in the past, and that this past moment differs significantly from the circumstance of the present, it can add a rational perspective to the emotional overwhelm. Remember, setting boundaries isn't about being mean—it's about taking care of yourself, which is essential, because you are the only person in this entire world that is solely in control of taking care of you.

2. Start Small

If the idea of setting boundaries feels overwhelming, start with smaller ones. Practice saying "no" to minor requests or expressing a simple preference. For example, if someone suggests a plan that doesn't work for you, politely decline and suggest an alternative instead of agreeing just to avoid the temporary discomfort of conflict.

After all, avoiding that momentary discomfort of conflict only results in an elongated discomfort of doing something that you never wanted to do in the first place.

Either way, you are uncomfortable, but one discomfort gets easier with practice while the other will progressively wear you out overtime and lead to resentment of those you love the most, to no fault of their own. The small victories of saying 'no' to little things will build your confidence over time and eventually you will be a boundary setting master.

3. Reframe Your Thinking

Instead of viewing boundaries as a source of conflict, see them as a form of self-respect. Setting boundaries is not about pushing people away; it's about creating healthy relationships where both parties feel respected and understood. Think of it this way: boundaries are like the bumper lanes in bowling—they help keep the game going smoothly without anyone veering too far off course (and if you are as bad at bowling as I am, they are absolutely necessary).

4. Role-Play Scenarios ... ok not the role play you are thinking.
If you're worried about how someone will react to your boundary, try role-playing the scenario. This can be done with a friend, therapist, or even in front of a mirror. Practising what you want to say can make the real conversation less intimidating. Plus, it gives you a chance to refine your approach so that you can express your needs clearly and calmly.

5. Accept Discomfort
Let's be real—setting boundaries can be uncomfortable, especially if you're not used to it. But just like a workout, a little discomfort can lead to growth. Remind yourself that it's okay to feel uneasy and that the discomfort is temporary. Over time, what once felt difficult will become natural.

6. Focus on the Benefits
Think about the positive outcomes that come from setting boundaries. More time for yourself, reduced stress, healthier relationships—these are all rewards for stepping out of your comfort zone. It's like trading a scratchy sweater for one that fits just right—it might take some getting used to, but the comfort is worth it.

7. Give Yourself Grace
Remember that setting boundaries is a skill, and like any skill, it takes practice. You might fumble, second-guess yourself, or even backtrack at times—and that's okay. Progress, not perfection, is the goal. Celebrate your efforts, no matter how small, and keep moving forward.
Setting boundaries is about valuing yourself enough to say, "This is what I need." It's not selfish; it's self-care. While it might feel awkward or scary at first, with practice, it will become an empowering tool that helps you navigate life with more confidence and ease.

Stress: Sex

Go ahead, put up that fence around your garden—you deserve to flourish in a space that's truly your own. Now that we have discussed how to set boundaries, here are some ideas of boundaries themselves:

1. **Know Your Limits:** Take time to understand what you are comfortable with and what you are not. It's ok to take things slowly and to change your mind at any time.

2. **Communicate Clearly:** Express your boundaries to your partner in a calm and clear manner. Use "I" statements to communicate your feelings and needs, such as "I feel uncomfortable when..." or "I need..."

3. **Listen to Your Gut:** Trust your instincts. If something doesn't feel right, it probably isn't. It's ok to stop or say no if you feel uncomfortable at any point.

4. **Seek Mutual Consent:** Ensure that both you and your partner are enthusiastically consenting to everything that happens. Consent is an ongoing process, and it should be reaffirmed regularly.

5. **Be Firm and Respectful:** Be firm in your boundaries and respect your partner's boundaries as well. Mutual respect is key to a healthy and safe sexual relationship.

7. **Revisit and Revise:** Boundaries can change over time. Make sure to revisit and discuss them regularly with your partner to ensure that you're both comfortable and on the same page.

Stress: Sex

Let's foster a culture where respect and consent are the norms. By talking openly about sex, we reduce its taboo, leading to healthier and more respectful interactions. For those of us who have experienced sexual assault, knowing and setting our boundaries becomes even more vital. Teaching young women about their right to say "no" is essential—not just to protect themselves but to empower them to make choices that feel right for them.

Sex can be a positive and enriching experience when approached with care and respect. It's okay to set boundaries and prioritise your safety. These actions don't just protect you; they empower you to enjoy sexual experiences on your terms. Remember, it's absolutely ok to say "no" whenever you need to. You are not responsible for managing anyone else's emotions, and you should never feel obligated to sacrifice your own comfort just to avoid a bit of awkwardness. Please my love, feel empowered to say "No".

Let's continue to support each other in these conversations. By doing so, we're not only fostering a safer environment but also empowering each other to embrace our natural desires in a way that feels right and safe. You deserve to feel confident, respected, and cherished in all your relationships. Let's work together to create a world where these values are the standard.

The Positive Side of Sex: Hormones and Their Impact

Oxytocin, affectionately known as the "love hormone," plays a significant role in sexual behaviour. A 2021 analysis concluded that orgasms can induce oxytocin, which in turn increases arousal and sexual desire. Beyond romantic connection, oxytocin is crucial in regulating social behaviour and reducing stress, blood pressure, and anxiety.

Stress: Sex

It's created by your hypothalamus, the brain's "office manager" of hormones, and stored in your posterior pituitary gland. This hormone enhances social interactions, making you feel more connected and less stressed. **Alternate activities that stimulate oxytocin:**

1. Positive Social Interactions

- **Spending Time with Loved Ones:** Engaging in meaningful conversations or activities with friends and family helps release oxytocin.
- **Acts of Kindness:** Doing something nice for someone, like giving a compliment or helping with a task, can increase oxytocin for both the giver and receiver.
- **Eye Contact:** Maintaining warm, friendly eye contact can also boost oxytocin levels, enhancing feelings of trust and connection.

2. Petting Animals

- **Interacting with Pets:** Petting, playing with, or even just spending time with animals can increase oxytocin, benefiting both humans and pets.

3. Mindfulness and Relaxation

- **Meditation:** Certain forms of meditation, especially those focusing on compassion and loving-kindness, can increase oxytocin levels.
- **Breathing Exercises:** Deep, slow breathing, particularly when done mindfully, can help release oxytocin and promote relaxation.

4. **Listening to Music**

- **Music Therapy:** Listening to music you love, especially with others, can stimulate the release of oxytocin, enhancing feelings of happiness and connection.

5. **Eating with Others**

- **Shared Meals:** Eating with others, especially in a relaxed and enjoyable setting, can lead to the release of oxytocin, fostering a sense of community and belonging.

6. **Exercise**

- **Group Activities:** Engaging in physical activities like yoga, dancing, or group sports with others can help boost oxytocin.
- **Endurance Exercises:** Long-duration activities like running, swimming, or cycling can increase oxytocin levels, particularly when done in nature or with others.

7. **Creative Expression**

- **Art and Crafting:** Participating in creative activities like painting, knitting, or any form of artistic expression, especially in a social setting, can stimulate oxytocin release.

8. **Laughing**

- **Humour and Laughter:** Sharing a good laugh with others can increase oxytocin levels, improving mood and social bonds.

9. Giving Gifts

- **Thoughtful Gifts:** Giving or receiving a thoughtful gift, even a small one, can enhance feelings of connection and trigger the release of oxytocin.

10. Supporting Others

- **Emotional Support**:** Being there for someone in need, offering a listening ear or a shoulder to cry on, can significantly increase oxytocin for both the giver and receiver.

Each of these activities not only boosts oxytocin but also contributes to overall emotional well-being and strengthens relationships. By regularly engaging in these practices, you can enhance your sense of connection, reduce stress, and improve your mental health .

Endorphins, particularly Beta-Endorphins, are your body's natural painkillers and mood elevators. These little guys are synthesised and stored in the anterior pituitary gland. They're released in response to stress, including during sex, exercise, and other activities. Endorphins block pain receptors and trigger the release of dopamine, the "feel-good" hormone. This can lead to what's often referred to as a "runner's high" during exercise, and a similar euphoric feeling during and after sex. Engaging in activities that release endorphins can help boost mood and emotional stability. This feel good cocktail is why it is crucial to select the person that you have sex with mindfully. Once endorphins and oxytocin are running the show, logic and reason (along with the ability to register red flags) is quick to go out the door.

Stress: Sex

Alternate activities that stimulate Endorphins:

1. Exercise

- **Cardio Workouts:** Activities like running, swimming, cycling, or aerobics are famous for triggering the "runner's high," a euphoric feeling caused by a rush of endorphins.
- **High-Intensity Interval Training (HIIT):** Short bursts of intense exercise followed by rest periods can also boost endorphin levels.
- **Strength Training:** Lifting weights or engaging in resistance training exercises can stimulate endorphin release.

2. Laughter

- **Watching Comedy:** Spending time watching a funny movie, TV show, or stand-up comedy can significantly increase endorphin levels.
- **Socialising with Friends:** Engaging in light-hearted, fun conversations with friends can lead to spontaneous laughter, boosting endorphins.

3. Music and Dancing:

- **Listening to Uplifting Music:** Enjoying your favourite tunes, especially ones that make you feel good, can help release endorphins.
- **Dancing:** Whether you're at a party or just dancing around your living room, moving to the rhythm can increase endorphin levels.

4. **Eating Certain Foods**

- **Spicy Foods:** Eating foods with like chilli peppers can cause a mild pain response in your mouth, leading to the release of endorphins.
- **Dark Chocolate:** Consuming dark chocolate can stimulate the production of endorphins, contributing to that feel-good sensation.

5. **Meditation and Yoga**

- **Mindfulness Meditation:** Regular meditation can increase endorphins, helping to reduce stress and improve mood.
- **Yoga:** The combination of physical postures, breath control, and meditation in yoga can boost endorphin levels, particularly in practices like Vinyasa or Ashtanga.

6. **Acupuncture**

- **Therapeutic Treatments:** Acupuncture, a traditional Chinese medicine practice, can stimulate endorphin release by targeting specific points on the body.

7. **Spending Time in Nature**

- **Hiking:** Walking in nature, especially in scenic environments, can promote the release of endorphins.
- **Sunlight Exposure:** Spending time outdoors in the sun can naturally boost endorphins, improving your mood.

8. Creative Activities

- **Art and Crafting:** Engaging in creative activities like painting, drawing, or knitting can help elevate endorphin levels.

- **Writing or Journaling:** Expressing your thoughts and emotions through writing can be a cathartic process, leading to the release of endorphins.

9. Volunteering and Helping Others

- **Acts of Kindness:** Helping others or volunteering can create a sense of purpose and fulfillment, which in turn boosts endorphin levels.

10. Enduring Cold Exposure

- **Cold Showers:** Taking a cold shower or plunge can shock the system and trigger endorphin release, leaving you feeling invigorated.

- **Cryotherapy:** This therapeutic technique involves brief exposure to extremely cold temperatures and is known to stimulate endorphin production.

11. Breathing Exercises

- **Deep Breathing Techniques:** Practices like pranayama or deep, diaphragmatic breathing can help calm the nervous system and increase endorphin levels.

Incorporating these activities into your routine can help naturally boost your endorphin levels, leading to improved mood, reduced pain, and an overall sense of well-being.

Stress: Sex

What I Wish I Had Known When I Was 16...

Ok - real talk. Using sex as a way to get someone to like you is like using a hammer to hang a picture—sure, it might get the job done, but it's a blunt tool, and the outcome is rarely as pretty as you hoped.

You're fabulous, full stop. If someone's into you, it should be for all the glorious, unique things that make you, well, you. Sex is amazing—when it's consensual, safe, and something you genuinely want to do. But here's the kicker: it's not a bargaining chip to win someone's affection. If you're hoping that hopping into bed will make them fall head over heels, you're setting yourself up for a disappointing sequel to a rom-com that never quite gets to the happy ending.

Sure, sex can make things feel intense, fast. It's like adding hot sauce to your relationship burrito—things heat up, and suddenly, it all feels a bit more exciting. But, much like hot sauce, if the only thing keeping you together is the spice, you're going to run out of steam (and maybe milk) pretty quickly.

You deserve someone who sees you as a whole person—not just a late-night booty call. The kind of relationship that stands the test of time is built on mutual respect, shared interests, and a connection that runs deeper than a few steamy nights. Think of sex as the cherry on top of an already delicious sundae, not the entire dessert.

Spoiler alert: There's no cheat code for making someone like you.
If someone's going to fall for you, it'll be because of your wit, your kindness, your ability to quote obscure 90s sitcoms at just the right moment—basically, all the things that make you the amazing person that you are beneath the surface. Sex doesn't fast-track this process.

Stress: Sex

It's more like adding a plot twist before you've really established the characters. You are worth more than just your ability to please someone in bed. If someone doesn't see that, it's their loss—not yours. Remember, sex should be something you want to do, not something you feel you *have* to do for you to keep someone around. If they're truly into you, they'll stick around for the whole story, not just the steamy chapters. Embrace your worth, hold out for the real deal, and never forget that you're more than enough just as you are.

What do you do if someone is lacking interest?
Understand that it's not about you. Someone else's lack of interest or inconsistency is about their emotional state, current capacity, preconceived and often subconscious beliefs, not your worth.
What works for them is up to them, your job is not to convince someone to love you, but to decide whether or not the way that they love, works for you. Someone else's behaviour, is **not** a reflection of your worth. **Your** behaviour and integrity is what defines you.
I used to use sex as a way to feel validated and it ultimately led to feelings of emptiness and a lack of connection. I now personally choose to not have sex outside of a committed relationship, because that is what feels aligned to me.
Sex is something that is completely personal, whatever you choose and whoever you choose, please ensure that it is on your terms my love (and theirs) #mutualconsent.

Let go of trying to control another individual's decision making process and trying to analyse someone else (we have all been there, it's ok) and redirect your energy into understanding yourself. Recognise your value and don't settle for less. By doing so, you'll attract relationships that truly appreciate and respect you.

Stress: Sex

Sex is a natural and beautiful part of life. When approached with respect, clear boundaries, and open communication, it can enhance your well-being and deepen your connection. Prioritise your safety, trust your instincts, and remember that it's ok to say no at any time. Embrace your natural desires in a way that feels right for you, when you are ready and support others in doing the same. Together, we can create a world where everyone feels confident, respected, and cherished in their relationships.

Communicating openly about sex is crucial for removing stigma, fostering healthy relationships, and ensuring that sexual expression occurs in a consensual and positive environment. **Here are some strategies to facilitate open, healthy conversations about sex:**

1. Start with Education and Awareness

- **Normalise Conversations:** Begin by discussing sex in a factual and non-judgmental way. This can be done through education, whether in schools, at home, or through self-education. Understanding the basics of sexual health, consent, and respect is fundamental.
- **Correct Misinformation:** Address and dispel myths or misconceptions about sex. This includes challenging harmful stereotypes, debunking unrealistic portrayals of sex in media, and promoting a realistic understanding of sexual relationships.

2. Create a Safe Space for Discussion

- **Encourage Open Dialogue:** Foster an environment where questions about sex can be asked without shame or fear of judgement. Whether with a partner, in educational settings, or with friends, ensure that discussions about sex are met with respect and openness.

- **Set Boundaries:** It's essential to discuss and respect personal boundaries. This includes talking about what each person is comfortable with, both physically and emotionally, and ensuring that these boundaries are honoured.

3. Promote Consent as a Cornerstone

- **Emphasise the Importance of Consent:** Consent should be clear, enthusiastic, and ongoing. It's important to communicate openly about what both partners want and don't want, ensuring that consent is always present.

- **Discuss Scenarios:** Talk about what consent looks like in different situations. This can help people understand that consent isn't just about saying "yes" or "no" but about mutual understanding and respect throughout the entire sexual experience.

4. Model Healthy Communication

- **Use "I" Statements:**** When discussing sex, frame your feelings and desires using "I" statements to avoid sounding accusatory or critical. For example, "I feel comfortable when..." or "I'd like to try..."

- **Listen Actively:** Just as important as expressing your own needs is listening to your partner's. Make sure both parties feel heard and understood.

5. Discuss Emotions and Expectations

- **Talk About Emotional Needs:** Sex isn't just a physical act; it often involves emotional intimacy. Discuss what sex means to each person, including any emotional expectations or concerns.

- **Address Stigma Head-On:** Recognise and discuss any feelings of shame or stigma associated with sex. Addressing these feelings openly can help reduce their power and promote a healthier, more positive view of sex.

6. Seek Professional Guidance if Needed

- **Counselling and Therapy:** If discussing sex feels particularly difficult, or if there are deeper issues at play, seeking guidance from a therapist or counsellor can be helpful. They can provide tools for communication and help navigate complex feelings or past traumas.

7. Respect Privacy and Confidentiality

- **Private Conversations:** Ensure that discussions about sex are private and respectful of each person's confidentiality. This fosters trust and makes it easier to communicate openly.

- **Avoid Gossip:** Refrain from sharing intimate details about sexual experiences with others unless both partners are comfortable with it.

8. Encourage a Culture of Respect

- **Promote Mutual Respect:** A healthy sexual relationship is built on mutual respect. Encourage conversations that highlight the importance of respecting each other's desires, boundaries, and emotions.

Stress: Sex

By following these strategies, we can shift the conversation around sex from one of stigma and suppression to one of openness, respect, and healthy expression. This not only fosters better individual relationships but also contributes to a more informed and empathetic society.

Stress: Sense of Self

This feels like the perfect time to introduce the self-love monster. You know the one—it's all over your Instagram feed, wrapped up in platitudes of "Love yourself first," "Be your own hero," and my personal favourite, "Focus on you, queen" — Cue the subtle eye roll.
Don't get me wrong—I'm not here to drag down the concept of self-care or independence. My issue is with how vague and mystical these messages can feel, as if self-love is some magical elixir you sip on when the stars align.

Once, at a self-actualisation workshop (yes, I went there), participants were asked to define the word love in 3-5 bullet points. Men, women, young, old—every single person had a wildly different answer. It hit me: how can we preach self-love when we can't even agree on what love itself means?
If we can't agree on love, how exactly are we supposed to "love" ourselves? To me, self-love often felt like the equivalent of trying to charge my laptop by plugging a USB into one side and a USB-C into the other—hoping for a miracle, only to stay exactly the same.

Take the Oxford Dictionary's stab at it: "an intense feeling of deep affection." By that logic, I suppose I'm in love with my satin pyjamas, but does that definition really encompass what we mean when we talk about love for family, friends, a partner or ourselves?
Love is everywhere, yet its meaning feels slippery—"unconditional love", "tough love", "in love,"—we use it all the time without really asking: what are we saying when we tell someone, "I love you"?

In my opinion, "deep affection" barely scratches the surface. Love encompasses gratitude, tenderness, compassion, and sometimes even sacrifice. Love is more than a word—it's a frequency, a commitment to act with the best intentions for yourself or another. But when it comes to self-love, how do we apply that frequency to ourselves without it sounding like one more item on the to-do list?

Recently, I came across a definition of self-love that stopped me in my tracks. In a video, Matthew Hussey compared self-love to the way a parent loves their child. Not because the child excels at maths or wears trendy clothes, but simply because "they're my child." What if we adopted that same unconditional care for ourselves? "I love myself simply because, I am my human." We've been given this body, this mind, and this life to nurture and protect—what more justification do we need to treat ourselves with care and respect?

But... How do we actually do it? The concept is sweet, sure, but what are the real, tangible steps we can take to cultivate this deep affection for ourselves? Let's be honest—treating ourselves with kindness often feels more like a bad comedy routine. High-fiving ourselves in the mirror? Awkward. Giving ourselves a pep talk? Cringe-worthy at best. But self-love doesn't have to feel so forced. It's about small, sustainable actions—ones that bring the abstract into the real. Let's dive into how to actually make this self-love thing work. Without the clichés. Without the fluff. Just practical steps to start showing up for yourself, as your own unwavering ally.

Stress: Sense of Self

1. Talk to Yourself Like You Would a Friend

Imagine your best friend is having a rough day, beating themselves up over a mistake. Would you scold them, or would you offer words of comfort and encouragement? (Hint: It's the latter.) Try to apply this same compassion to yourself. When you catch yourself spiralling into self-criticism, pause and reframe your thoughts as if you were speaking to a friend. It's the same as sending yourself a care package, except it's verbal, and you don't have to pay for postage.

2. Practice Mindfulness Without the Pretzel-Like Yoga Poses

You don't need to bend yourself into a pretzel or chant "om" for hours to be mindful—though this is fun and I recommend it when you have the time, it is not essential. Mindfulness simply means being present, to notice your thoughts and feelings without judgement. This can be as simple as taking a few deep breaths, acknowledging what you're feeling, and allowing the sensation to be there without over analysing it. It's as if you are having a casual chat with your inner self—no need for formalities, just a moment of awareness.

3. Write Yourself a Love Letter (Yes, Really)

Ok, this one might sound a bit twee, but hear me out. Writing a letter to yourself can be a powerful exercise in self-compassion. Instead of dwelling on what's wrong, focus on what you appreciate about yourself—your strengths, your resilience, the little things that make you, well, you. Think of it as a love letter to your future self, filled with all the affection and encouragement you'd want to hear on a bad day. Just remember to keep it in a safe place, away from prying eyes or the recycle bin.

Stress: Sense of Self

4. Set Boundaries

Ah, this old chest nut. Self-compassion isn't just about being kind to yourself; it's also about protecting your energy. Setting boundaries—whether it's saying no to extra work, carving out time for yourself, or distancing yourself from people that are toxic for you—shows that you value your own well-being. Think of it as drawing a line in the sand, not to keep others out, but to keep yourself in a safe and loving space.

5. Embrace Your Flaws with Grace

Perfection is overrated, and frankly, impossible. Embracing your flaws—whether it's a crooked smile, a tendency to procrastinate, or that awkward dance move you break out at every wedding—is a key part of self-compassion. Rather than viewing these quirks as negatives, see them as unique aspects of your character. It's like finding a chipped tea cup in an antique store—its imperfections make it all the more charming.

6. Give Yourself Permission to Feel

Emotions can be messy, unpredictable, and downright inconvenient, but they're also an essential part of being human. Give yourself permission to feel without judgement—whether you're sad, angry, anxious, or just plain tired. Allowing yourself to experience emotions fully is a radical act of self-compassion. It's the equivalent of giving yourself a hall pass for being human—no detention necessary.

7. Rest

Stop treating yourself as a machine and take rest when your body needs it. This also requires paying close enough attention to your body to signals to acknowledge when that time for rest arrives, and then relentlessly honouring that.

Stress: Sense of Self

8. Treat Yourself to a Self-Care Ritual

Think of self-care as a way to show yourself some love in a tangible, practical way. Whether it's a bubble bath, a quiet walk in nature, or even just five minutes of stretching before bed, find a ritual that nourishes you. This isn't about indulgence for indulgence's sake, but rather about giving yourself what you need to recharge. It's like giving yourself a mini vacation, minus the travel stress and sunburn.

In the end, self-compassion isn't about being perfect or having all the answers. It's about being gentle with yourself, accepting your humanity, and finding ways to show yourself the love and care that you so freely give to others. Because let's be honest, life is a much nicer experience when you honour your own needs.

Purpose.

Purpose

Purpose, according to the Oxford Dictionary, is the reason why something is done, created, or exists. It's like the cosmic nudge that drags you out of bed in the morning, even when your blanket has a death grip on you. The Cambridge Dictionary, trying to sound equally sophisticated, describes it as an intention or aim—a reason for doing something or for letting something happen. Pretty fancy definitions, right? But let's break it down.

Imagine purpose as your personal GPS, only instead of recalculating when you miss a turn, it steers your life decisions, shapes your goals, and keeps you from ending up in existential traffic. For some, purpose is all about their career—finding that dream job that's as satisfying as the first sip of coffee on a Monday morning. For others, it's about the people they love, or even a hobby that sparks more joy than a perfectly executed TikTok dance.

William Damon, a researcher who penned "A Path to Purpose" takes it up a notch (Glazer, 2008). He defines purpose as "a stable and generalised intention to accomplish something that is meaningful to the self and consequential for the world beyond the self". Translation: it's about doing something that not only lights up your life but also brightens up the world a little bit. Think of it like adding sprinkles to a cupcake—you're sweetening your own existence while making everything around you a tad more delightful.

Whether your purpose is curing diseases, raising tiny humans, or perfecting the art of sourdough, just remember—it's your North Star, guiding you through the maze of life, even when the road gets bumpy or the Wi-Fi signal of your soul gets a little weak.

Purpose: Presence

Having a purpose means knowing what you want to achieve and why it matters. Research shows that people with a sense of purpose are happier, more resilient, and more successful than those who don't have one. Purpose isn't a one-size-fits-all. It can be a career goal, a personality trait, or even small daily acts like smiling at a stranger or complimenting your barista. Only you can define your purpose in life.

For me, purpose hit home during a conversation that I had with my dad when I was the ripe old age of nine years old. We were driving somewhere insignificant when I blurted out, "Dad, what's the meaning of life?" Without missing a beat, he said, "To make the best choice you can in each moment. Live each moment to the best of your ability, and you'll lead a beautiful life."

So, how do we make the best decision in each moment? That's where presence comes in. Initially, I called this section "Purpose, Productivity, and Perspective" but I swapped productivity for presence because being busy doesn't always mean you're living a fulfilled life.
Sometimes, productivity becomes a distraction from life itself.

I've been guilty of obsessing over productivity, often at the expense of enjoying life. No time for breaks or connection when there's a to-do list to conquer. But what's the point of achieving a lot if you're missing out on life's little joys? Productivity can exist without purpose, but presence cannot, because presence is the purpose of life itself. Every moment spent being fully present is a moment spent productively.
The ability to be present is closely tied to acceptance. Accepting life as it is and finding peace in each moment. Remember, 99% of the harm is in our minds; only 1% is the actual situation itself. By focusing on the present, we can feel more at home in our mind and body, reconnecting

with this wild experience that we call life.
Alright, let's dive into the wonderland of perspective with a fresh twist! Imagine it as trying on a pair of designer shades—not just any old pair, but the kind that makes everything look a little sharper, a bit more glamorous, and gives you that "I've got this" vibe. A simple shift in perspective can totally flip your life experience, like switching from black-and-white to full Technicolor. It's like listening to your favourite song—when you're in a good mood, it's an anthem, but when you're feeling down, even the happiest tune sounds off-key.

The key thing to remember is that you're always the one holding the remote. You have the power to change the channel, adjust the volume, or even switch to a new playlist altogether. You've got an entire wardrobe of perspectives at your disposal, and you get to decide which one to strut out in.

Every perspective has its ups and downs. Sometimes, slipping into a "victim" mindset feels like wrapping yourself in a cosy blanket of self-pity. It's tempting because it might attract sympathy, like getting a free pass to the pity party. But let's be honest—it's a bit like handing the keys to your life over to someone else and hoping they don't crash it. It's comforting for a moment, sure, but long term? It's like letting someone else drive your dream car, and they don't even know how to parallel park.

Taking responsibility for your life is like getting back behind the wheel, saying, "Nope, I've got this!" It's empowering because it means you're choosing the destination. You're setting the GPS to where you want to go—whether it's towards positive changes, better relationships, or setting those healthy boundaries. You're not just a passenger; you're the

driver, the navigator, and the DJ.
Owning your life also comes with a bonus: self-awareness. It's akin to finding the secret manual to your own brain. Suddenly, you start to understand the patterns, see the triggers, and know exactly what makes you tick. It's like unlocking a cheat code that lets you boost your happiness, calm your stress, and max out your potential. Plus, there's something pretty satisfying about knowing you're the one making it all happen.

Perspective isn't just a way to keep your cool when life throws curveballs; it's your secret weapon for bouncing back. When things go sideways—and they inevitably will—your perspective can either make you feel like you've failed spectacularly or like you've just collected another badge of wisdom. Take, for example, the time I got fired from a job in my first week. Not exactly a highlight reel moment, but I knew it was because I was completely underqualified for what was expected of me in that role. Instead of wallowing, I quickly reassured myself that getting the boot was the best thing that could have happened. My short lived experience in the job opened my eyes to a new interest in graphic design and it pointed me in the right direction. Within 24 hours of losing that job, I was enrolled in a course, found an interim job and the new found flexibility also allowed me to make a move to a new destination that I otherwise wouldn't have had the freedom to do. If I had stayed in that job, I would be making a quarter of the wage that I do now, only a few years later and I wouldn't be writing my own book, I can tell you that much.

By taking full responsibility for my reaction, I felt empowered, resilient, and optimistic about the future. You always have a choice—one path might make you feel like you're stuck in quicksand, while the other makes you feel like a wise old sage collecting wisdom points.

Purpose: Perspective

Choosing a positive perspective can turn challenges into opportunities. That tough maths test? It's not a nightmare; it's a chance to prove how much you've learned. Even if you fail, it's feedback, not a final verdict. And hey, if it all goes horribly wrong, at least it makes for a great story later! Plus, perspective is the secret sauce in your relationships. Instead of seeing a sibling's annoying habit as a reason to argue, you might start to appreciate their quirky charm. Perspective can turn conflicts into bonding moments and everyday annoyances into opportunities for connection. From now on, think of your perspective as the ultimate accessory—it can make life's ups and downs more manageable, turn ordinary moments into epic adventures, and keep you connected with the people who matter most.

While we are on the topic of perspective, let's throw a new lens on our approach to self blame. There is a big difference between taking responsibility and opting for self blame, one enables you to take control of your life while the other makes it hard to get out of bed in the morning. Navigating self-blame with the additional information that hindsight so generously offers can often feel a bit like trying to untangle Christmas lights—frustrating, time-consuming, and sometimes you're not even sure why you bothered in the first place. But, instead of tossing those lights (or your feelings) out the window, let's take a deep breath and approach this with a little bit of self compassion.

Self blame is that sneaky voice in your head, a bit like a terrible backseat driver, constantly reminding you of how you *could* have taken a different route. But here's the thing: you made the best decision that you could with the information you had at the time. Hindsight is a bit of a know-it-all, but it's important to remember that you didn't have the luxury of that perspective when you made your choices.

Purpose: Perspective

Regret is like getting ghosted by someone you thought was "the one"—it stings, it's confusing, and you're left replaying every moment, wondering what went wrong. But what if I told you that this heartbreak is actually setting the stage for something better? Just like how the universe has a way of clearing out the wrong people to make room for the right ones, regret often signals that there's a lesson or a new opportunity on the horizon. You might not see it now, but one day, you'll look back and realise that the choice you regret today was actually steering you toward a future you wouldn't trade for anything.

And now, onto that pesky hindsight. It's easy to look back and think, "Well, duh, I should have seen that coming". The truth is, life isn't a well-written sitcom where everything wraps up neatly in 30 minutes. It's more like improv comedy—unscripted, unpredictable, and sometimes downright frustrating. Embrace that unpredictability as part of your journey. You're not a character in a TV show; you're a human being doing your best. Sometimes you will feel like you have made the wrong choice, but it was the right choice, in that moment, and now with more information, you can make a different decision.
The key is to treat yourself with the same kindness that you would offer a friend. If your best mate told you that they were stuck in a cycle of self-blame, you wouldn't tell them to keep dwelling on it, would you? No, you'd probably hand them a cup of tea (or something stronger) and remind them that they're only human. Do yourself a favour and extend that same kindness inward.

Instead of letting hindsight bully you into feeling bad about the past, use it as a guide to make better decisions moving forward. Think of it as a rearview mirror: useful for seeing where you've been, but not something you should be staring at while trying to drive forward.

Purpose: Perspective

Remember, life is full of lessons, albeit sometimes annoying ones—some are learned in the moment, and some take a little time (and maybe a few extra mistakes) to sink in. Next time self-blame comes knocking, greet it with a knowing smile, maybe a witty one-liner, and the understanding that you are doing the best that you can with the wisdom you've gained along the way.

New lens for Regret:

Regret is a life lesson with a stubborn agenda—it was going to teach you, one way or another. Think of it as the universe's way of saying, "You needed this, and if it wasn't now, it would have been later, probably in a worse scenario". The key here is to understand that this lesson was inevitable. Instead of dwelling on what could have been, dive deep into the experience and extract every ounce of wisdom it has to offer, ensuring you don't have to sit through this class again.

Life is full of stumbles, and while you will inevitably fall, what matters is that you know how to get back up.

Regret often stems from the fact that you made the best decision you could at the time, given the information that you had. Forgive yourself for not being able to predict the future—after all, you're not a psychic, or at least not a good one–you are just a human being trying to navigate this unpredictable world.

Here's your prescription mantra: "I forgive myself for not knowing what the future held and for making the best decision that I could at the time to give myself what I needed at that moment". Now, to truly move on, ask yourself: What do I need to learn from this to let it go? If all else fails, think of regret like poop. Yes, you read that right. It's an inevitable part of life that, if held onto, will only give you a bellyache. But once you let it go? Instant relief, and you feel ten times lighter.

Purpose: Perspective

New lens on the unpredictability of life:
Life's unpredictability is like trying to master the perfect winged eyeliner—just when you think you've nailed it, one side decides to go rogue, and suddenly you're rocking an accidental Cleopatra look. The first step to embracing this chaos is to recognise that life isn't a polished highlight reel. It's more like a series of Instagram Stories: unfiltered, full of surprises, and often more relatable when things don't go as planned.

Instead of stressing about what's around the corner (spoiler: it's probably something you didn't plan for), try treating life like the improv show that we spoke about earlier. When the unexpected happens, say "yes, and..." rather than "no, but..." It's about flowing with the plot rather than trying to rewrite the script on the fly. Remember, it's ok to not have all the answers, because half the fun is figuring things out as you go.

Picture yourself as a ship's captain, steering through the stormy seas of life. The weather? Completely out of your control. The ocean currents? Yep, not your department. But the way you navigate, the direction you choose, and how tightly you grip the wheel—that's all you.
External control is the mirage in the desert of chaos. We like to think that if we just try hard enough, we can control the outcome of every situation. Spoiler alert: we cannot.
What we can control is our response, our attitude, and our decisions in the face of whatever life throws at us. Think of internal stability as your emotional anchor. No matter how wild the seas get, it keeps you grounded, steady, and prevents you from capsizing when things don't go as planned. The human brain is a bit like a dog with a chew toy—it loves gnawing on problems, especially the ones it can't quite sink its teeth into. And when it can't solve the problem, it just keeps chewing, creating an endless loop of worry, stress, and "what-ifs."

Purpose: Perspective

Here's a concept that might help break that loop:
"Let go or be dragged."

Sometimes, the brain needs a reminder that not every problem is yours to solve, not every puzzle piece fits perfectly, not every question has an answer and needing an answer is just latching onto that previously spoken about illusion of being able to control external circumstances. Imagine trying to teach a cat to fetch. It's a noble effort, but ultimately, you're going to end up frustrated while the cat stares at you like you've lost your mind. Similarly, trying to make sense of someone else's behaviour or a situation beyond your control is like chasing that elusive cat—you're better off letting go and focusing on what you can manage. The next time you catch yourself spiralling into a thought loop, take a deep breath and ask, "Is this my cat to chase?" If the answer is no, set it down, walk away, and give your brain something else to chew on—preferably something that doesn't involve an existential crisis.

In life, no choice is inherently 'right' or 'wrong.' The secret is not in the choice itself but in how we navigate its inevitable twists and turns. Every path, whether glamorous or mundane, will deliver its share of peaks and valleys. What remains constant is that, regardless of the road chosen, you're destined to encounter the full range of human emotions. That's the core of existence: not in the pursuit of a perfect life, but in savouring every imperfect moment of it.

Attention.

Attention

Alright, let's dive into something that can really level up your life—training your attention. We just chatted about purpose, presence, and perspective. All of these require a bit of finesse when it comes to where you direct your attention. So, let's talk about mindfulness.

Mindfulness is a mental spa day where you focus on the present, deliberately and without judgement. This practice can help you stay calm and collected, even in the middle of a stress storm. Plus, it's fantastic for your mental health, reducing stress, and improving sleep. Mindfulness can take many forms—meditation, breathwork, body scans, journaling, yoga, qigong, walking in nature, sitting in nature, mindful eating, or just unplugging from your phone for a bit to hang out with yourself, sounds wild right?

You've probably heard someone say, "enjoy every moment, life is short". You might have rolled your eyes at your well-meaning relative, but guess what? There's some serious truth to it. Mindfulness is all about being fully aware of what's happening right now—what's going on inside you and around you. It means not living life on autopilot but actually experiencing each moment as it unfolds. When the present moment shifts towards the painful side of life, we may feel an aversion to experiencing it. It is important to remember that pain is just as important as happiness, it is simply a guide that helps us navigate towards living a meaningful and aligned life.

Dr. Margaret Chesney from the University of California, San Francisco, is studying the significant impact that mindfulness can have on our health. She notes that, what is valuable about mindfulness is that it is accessible, anytime, anywhere (Mindfulness Matters, 2017).

Attention

One study found a link between mindfulness meditation and changes in brain regions involved in memory, learning, and emotion. Another study showed that mindfulness might reduce anxiety and hostility among urban youth, leading to less stress, fewer fights, and better relationships.

One of the coolest things about mindfulness is how it encourages you to pay attention to your thoughts, actions, and body. For example, mindful eating can help people maintain a healthy weight. Instead of munching mindlessly in front of the TV, you eat when you're hungry, savour each bite, and stop when you're full. Often the most simple strategies are the most effective, but they are easier said than done.
Sure, fitting mindfulness into our fast-paced lives can be a challenge. We love multitasking and speeding through endless to-do lists (speaking for myself here). The truth is, mindfulness enhances productivity and efficiency. 10 minutes in your morning can transform how you act through your entire day. It is one of the only investments that you can make in life with a guaranteed positive ROI.

You can practise mindfulness anytime—while answering emails, sitting in traffic, or waiting in line. Become aware of your breath, your feet on the ground, your fingers typing, and the people around you. I find that checking in with each of my senses, one by one can really help bring my mind back to the now. As you practise, you'll notice how much your mind races to the past or future - that's ok! Gently nudge your mind back to the present moment, these little steps add up, creating a more mindful and healthy life.

Attention: Acceptance

For me, mindfulness means continuously bringing my attention back to my breath throughout the day. I check in with myself: How am I breathing? Is it slow and calm, or fast and restricted? If it's the latter, why? I discovered I was often stressed without even realising it, completely unaware that my breathing was short or almost non-existent. By regularly checking in with my breath, I've become more aware of how everyday situations can impact my nervous system. This awareness has allowed me to re-train my response to stress by maintaining calm, slow breathing.

Before you roll your eyes and lump mindfulness in with kale smoothies and crystal healing, give it a shot. It's that thing you swore you'd never try but secretly loved—only this time, instead of guilty pleasure, it's about feeling more present, relaxed, and in control.

Attention: Acceptance

Next topic of conversation is a fun one, acceptance.
Picture this: life is a giant game of dodgeball, sometimes you're dodging the balls like a pro, other times you're getting smacked right in the face. Practicing acceptance is putting on an invisible suit of armour that lets you laugh off the hits and stay in the game with a smile.
Acceptance isn't about being a doormat or settling for less. It's about recognising that some things are out of your control, and that's completely ok. Imagine trying to stop a thunderstorm by yelling at the sky—hysterical, right? Accepting that you can't control the weather lets you grab an umbrella and dance in the rain instead.

Day to day, acceptance can save you from a ton of unnecessary stress. Your favourite coffee shop runs out of your go-to latte? Instead of letting it ruin your morning, accept it and try a new drink. Who knows, you might discover a new favourite! Traffic jams, surprise tests, or your little brother's non-stop Fortnite commentary—all become less irritating when you practice acceptance. It's your secret superpower that keeps you cool, calm, and collected.

Here's the deal: resistance is futile. Fighting against what you can't change, is the equivalent to trying to hold back the ocean with a mop —trust me, I have tried. You end up tired, wet, and cranky. When you practice acceptance, you conserve your energy for the things you can change —your attitude, your actions, and your choices. It's all about rolling with the punches and finding your groove. Let's not forget the mental health perks. Acceptance helps you manage stress and anxiety because you're not constantly battling reality, giving your brain a well-deserved vacation. When you stop fighting against what is and start accepting it, you free up headspace for creativity, joy, and, let's be honest, binge-watching your favourite shows without guilt.

Here's a cheeky bonus: acceptance can make you a total zen master. People will wonder how you stay so chill in the face of chaos. Your secret? You've mastered the art of going with the flow. Accepting life as it comes makes you more adaptable and resilient. You become like a bamboo tree, bending with the wind but never breaking.

Next time life throws you a curveball, mindfully practice acceptance. Embrace the unexpected, laugh at the absurd, and remember that acceptance is your ticket to a smoother, happier ride. Life's a game of dodgeball, and with acceptance, you're in for one heck of a fun match!

Please note: acceptance is NOT suppression or false positivity. It's allowing, comfortable and uncomfortable emotions to be there. This too shall pass.

Community.

I swapped judging and criticising others for a compassionate tone of voice and suddenly found that this shift flowed into how I spoke to myself too.

I stopped blaming others if I became triggered and instead asked myself, where is this trigger coming from? What part of me is bothered by this?

I understand now that anytime I look to fix or change others, I am really just trying to avoid addressing something deeper within myself.

Community

Imagine your life as a meticulously curated art gallery. Each relationship, experience, and moment is a piece on display, contributing to the overall narrative of who you are. Alone, a single piece might be intriguing, but when you step back, you realise the true power lies in the collective—the connections between them, the interplay of perspectives, the rich tapestry that emerges when they're all viewed together.

Being part of a community is having an exclusive membership to this gallery, where everyone is both a curator and a contributor. It's not just about belonging; it's about being part of something larger that enhances your personal collection, making the whole exhibit more profound and meaningful. It turns out, this isn't just a lofty metaphor; the benefits of being in a community were a significant focus of our studies at the Institute of Integrative Nutrition. Connectedness doesn't just elevate your spirits—it has tangible effects on lowering stress, boosting your immune system, and potentially adding years to your life. Who knew your social circle could be as essential as your morning vitamins?

When it comes to support, your community acts like the conservation team for your gallery. They're there to help restore your sense of well-being when life's wear and tear starts to show. Studies show that social support can help you bounce back faster from setbacks, after a particularly tough day, they're the ones who can help you view your challenges through a new lens, providing a fresh unseen perspective. Surrounding yourself with a community that shares your values and goals is filling your gallery with masterpieces instead of second-rate prints. It elevates the entire experience, inspiring you to aim higher and achieve more, all while making your ambitions feel not just possible, but inevitable.

Community

Let's not forget the joy that community brings. Think of those moments of spontaneous connection, the shared laughter that echoes through the gallery halls, turning ordinary days into memorable ones. Those are the moments that add depth and colour to your life's exhibit, making the experience richer and more fulfilling.

On a deeper level, community gives your life context. Just as every great gallery has a theme or story, the connections you make and the support that you give and receive add layers of meaning to your own story. Whether you're helping someone through a tough time or simply being present for a friend, these interactions give your life substance, like the purposeful brushstrokes that bring a painting to life.

Building and maintaining your community is like expanding your gallery's collection. It takes effort, sure, but the rewards are immeasurable. I know that for me personally, what I am doing or where I am is kind of irrelevant, as long as I have good people around me. I can work in a job that I don't love that much if I have good people, I can stay somewhere mediocre if I am surrounded by good people. We discussed earlier that presence is the purpose of life, the ability to be fully present is also the foundation for fostering deep and meaningful connections. Reach out, invest time, and cultivate those relationships. Whether you're joining a new group or deepening existing connections, each step enhances the richness of your life.

In the end, a strong community is your gallery's secret weapon. It keeps you resilient, supported, and ensures that your life's collection is as vibrant and diverse as possible. Cherish those connections, and remember: life's a gallery, and every piece has its place.

Community

Health benefits

The notion that community is woven into the very fabric of our existence isn't just a warm, fuzzy idea—it's firmly grounded in scientific evidence. Picture this: Relationships are the lattice of support, each connection weaving us into a tighter fabric of well-being. Steven Crane, a social engagement scholar at Stanford, puts it best: "Our relationships form the largest single factor in overall well-being. We need to prioritise showing up for one another because when we don't, loneliness and isolation become chronic" (Shetty, 2023).
In other words, if we start ghosting our social ties, we might as well start taking isolation as seriously as we take our skincare routines.

Let's discuss further, stress during isolation? It's not just a mood killer; it's a literal health hazard. The behaviours we adopt when we're cut off from others can make us more vulnerable to disease, and yes, even an earlier exit than planned. If that doesn't sound serious enough, the World Health Organization has officially placed social isolation up there with the big offenders: smoking, obesity, and elongated solo Netflix binges. On the upside, healthy social networks are a superpower, boosting your odds of long-term survival by a solid 50%.

Turns out, the longer we're isolated, the more our brains get stressed—like a computer overheating from too many open tabs. Prolonged stress tweaks our brain structure, creating havoc with the hypothalamic-pituitary-adrenal (HPA) axis. Remember that fancy thing, the body's chief operator that regulates everything from your nervous system to your immune response. Just like that dodgy Wi-Fi signal in a hotel lobby, chronic isolation messes with this essential pathway, leading to all sorts of long-term issues.

Community

Here's the kicker—those changes to the HPA axis are eerily similar to the impacts of adverse childhood events. That stress from being socially cut off? It's like reliving a drama from your past on repeat, impacting your emotional regulation and that feel-good factor of reward processing.

Areas involved in stress responses, the prefrontal cortex, amygdala, and hippocampus, start acting up, while regions such as the default mode network (DMN) shut down faster than your enthusiasm on a Monday morning. Acute loneliness gives us a desperate urge to connect, but chronic loneliness? That dims the desire for connection altogether, like a phone with its battery on 1%.

We are hardwired for connection, a design feature from evolution. The warm fuzzies you feel after a brunch with your closest pals? That's not just the mimosas talking; it's your brain getting actual neurological rewards. Positive social interactions light up brain pathways linked to motivation and reward. Getting someone to laugh? It's like receiving an internal applause from your neural circuits. These interactions are pure dopamine currency—is your brain getting five-star Uber ratings.

Now, about that A+ you got last week? Turns out you're more likely to cherish a night out celebrating with friends than the solo satisfaction of a high score. The science behind this is rooted in the brain's reward system, particularly within the corticostriatal circuits—the same pathways that light up when we experience pleasure or achieve a goal. When we recall positive social experiences, such as a night out with friends, these circuits are activated, much like when we receive a tangible reward. In essence, achieving your goals and then celebrating those victories with supportive people gives you a two-for-one deal... scientifically speaking.

Community

As for those feel-good vibes during social interactions, they're not just exclusive to humans. Even mice—yes, mice—experience an oxytocin-induced dopamine surge during their social gatherings, encouraging all kinds of prosocial behaviour. Who knew the mouse equivalent of a cheese and wine night could teach us something about the importance of connection?

The good news? Positive social connections have real survival benefits. We are talking, increase-your-odds-by-50% type of benefits. And even the perceived presence of a supportive friend, whether it's holding hands, seeing a familiar face, or even reading a note from a loved one, can lower stress responses. This is backed by both research and the life-long friendships of wild female baboons, who've figured out that social bonds reduce stress and improve longevity. Baboons: 1, Isolation: 0.

Even as we age, maintaining social connections becomes our brain's best defence against cognitive decline. Studies show that lonely adults' cognitive abilities decline up to 20% faster, whereas those with solid social networks preserve their mental health. Even weaker social ties can stave off depression. Whether it's your best friend or your favourite barista, those interactions might be keeping your brain sharper than a well-planned grocery list.

Social connection doesn't just keep us alive—it shapes our decisions. Take rodents, for example: they'd rather skip an addictive substance just to hang out with a friend. Translation? Sometimes, we choose real connection over unhealthy cravings. This could explain why support groups are so effective—they offer non-toxic substitutes for bad habits, kind of like swapping out vodka for kombucha at your next girls' night.

Community

Then there's the magic of shared experiences. Ever found yourself in sync with a friend while binge-watching a show? That's not just a coincidence—it's science. Sharing emotional experiences actually synchronises facial expressions, heart rates, and even how connected you feel to your viewing partner. The longer you interact, the deeper the connection becomes. Turns out, Netflix and chill isn't just a thing—it's a bonding ritual.

Finally, how do we know what someone else is thinking or feeling? Social interactions give us clues through tiny signals, like a smile or a generous gesture. These actions help us understand others' intentions, which strengthens our social bonds. We use empathy, theory of mind, and mentalizing—basically, understanding that others have their own thoughts and feelings—to stay connected. It's like adjusting your playlist to match the mood of the room: fine-tuning your social radar keeps you in sync with others, and that's where the magic happens.

Oh, and those dopamine hits you get from a friend's smile? They're not just fleeting moments of joy—they're your brain's way of reinforcing positive social connections. Go ahead and treasure that coffee date with your bestie; you're literally rewiring your brain for more happiness. As Steven Crane so simply puts it: "If you want a friend, be a friend" (Shetty, 2023). Kindness, it seems, is the best way to build connections—and building connections is the best way to build a life worth celebrating.

Community

Crafting Your Circle of Influence

"When was the last time this person genuinely brought joy into your life?"

Take a moment to mull over this. Do the people surrounding you make you feel secure, aligned with your values, and driven towards your goals?

There's a popular notion that you become the average of the five people you spend the most time with. While I have not personally scoured peer-reviewed journals to confirm this, it does circulate widely on Instagram reels from individuals with an air of authority—so it must have some merit, right?

Curating Your Inner Circle

- How do these individuals affect your emotional landscape?
- How do they steer your actions and decisions?
- Are they the wind beneath your wings or the anchor holding you back?

Community

A supportive community isn't just a luxury—it's a necessity.
The benefits are manifold:

- **Oxytocin Surge:** The love hormone, providing that warm, fuzzy feeling.
- **Cortisol Reduction:** Lowering the stress hormone that turns you into the proverbial grumpy cat.
- **Insulin Regulation:** Keeping your blood sugar—and mood—on an even keel.
- **Sex Hormone Balance:** Because everyone deserves a bit of hormonal harmony.

Community

The Art of Communication

Mastering the art of saying 'no' to what doesn't light you up—and resisting the urge to say 'yes' out of guilt.
Clear communication prevents misunderstandings, creating a much more tranquil existence for both yourself and those around you. Expressing your feelings rather than bottling them up can be transformative. It's not about being rude; it's about blending warmth, kindness, and honesty.

- **Detail Behaviour:** Replace vague accusations such as "you always" with specific statements, for example: "twice now, once last week and again yesterday."
- **Pause and Reflect:** Before reacting, take a moment to sit with your feelings. Ask yourself, What is bothering me about this situation?

Is this something that I need to address within myself or with someone else? For instance, instead of saying, "It's so annoying when you constantly call and text me," try, "I'm feeling quite stressed with my current workload and need some space. I appreciate your desire for contact and ask that I can reach out once I'm ready."

By communicating with clarity and non-violence, you can stand firm and self-assured. How others respond is beyond your control and often says more about them than you.
Clear communication will swiftly reveal who respects your boundaries and who is better kept at a polite distance.
People will love you, people will despise you, and most of the time, it will have little to do with you. We all operate from our own belief systems and conditioning. It's easier to shed beliefs that no longer serve you when you approach them with gentle curiosity.

Community

Not everyone is on that journey—some cling to their conditioning as if it defines them and it is important to remember that is their path, not yours.

If someone's communication style is detrimental to your well-being, you're well within your rights to walk away, no matter the circumstances. By establishing your safe space and setting firm boundaries, you empower yourself to lead a more serene and fulfilling life.

Community: Communication

Let's elaborate on the fancy science facts about connection—one of the most underrated superpowers for your physical, emotional, and mental health. Imagine you're a smartphone, what happens if you're not connected to Wi-Fi or a network? You're basically just a fancy paperweight. The same goes for us humans, connection keeps us charged, functional, and thriving.

First, let's look at physical health. People with strong social ties have lower rates of heart disease, better immune function, and even longer lifespans. It's like having a secret health elixir, only instead of being brewed by wizards, it's created through friendship. Just think: a hug from a friend can lower your blood pressure and reduce stress hormones. Basically what I am saying is, more hugs, less stress—that's science.

Next up, emotional health. Picture your emotions as a garden. Connection is like the sunlight and water that help your emotional flowers bloom. When you feel connected, you experience higher levels of happiness and lower levels of anxiety and depression. Sharing your feelings, laughing together, or even having a good cry with someone can act as emotional fertiliser, helping you grow and flourish. It's a spa day for your soul, without the hefty price tag.

Then there's mental health. Connection is like the ultimate brain workout. Engaging in conversations, sharing ideas, and even debating the best pizza toppings (cue debate re Pineapple on a pizza if you live in Australia) keep your mind sharp. Social interactions stimulate cognitive functions and can help protect against memory decline as you age. Plus, having a strong support system means you have people to help you navigate life's mental mazes.

Community: Communication

But wait, there's more! Connection also helps you build resilience. Life can throw some pretty hefty curveballs, and having a network of supportive people can help you catch those curveballs with grace (or at least not drop them on your foot). Knowing you have a support network to turn to makes you more adaptable and better equipped to handle stress. It's your mental and emotional safety net, always there to catch you when you need it most.

How do you tap into this powerful network of connections? Start by investing time in your relationships. Reach out to friends and family, join clubs or groups that interest you, and don't be afraid to meet new people. Engage in meaningful conversations, be present, and show genuine interest in others. By doing this, you are planting seeds of connection that will grow into a lush, supportive forest.

In a nutshell, connection is vital for your physical, emotional, and mental wellbeing. It keeps you happy, healthy and sharp as a knife (not a butter knife because they are relatively blunt when compared to other knives). My point is, make time for the people who matter, build those connections, and remember: life is better when we're all connected... and it's a lot more fun.

Community: Extra Notes

What to Look for in a Relationship: Dr. John Gottman's Five Essentials:

According to renowned relationship expert Dr. John Gottman, there are five key qualities you should look for in a partner to foster a strong, healthy relationship. These essentials create the foundation for long-term emotional connection and trust:

Honesty

A relationship must be built on trust, and that starts with honesty. Look for someone who is truthful, even when it's uncomfortable. A partner who doesn't lie gives you the security to be open and vulnerable, knowing you're operating in a space of mutual respect and trust.

Transparency

Transparency means they're willing to let you in. Whether it's sharing their thoughts, feelings, or past experiences, a transparent partner doesn't keep you guessing. They invite you into their inner world, and you feel welcome there, not like an outsider.

Accountability

This is about more than just making promises; it's about following through. A partner who holds themselves accountable for their actions demonstrates reliability and respect for your time and feelings. When they say they'll do something, they actually do it—this builds trust over time.

Community: Extra Notes

Ethical Actions

It's not enough for a partner to just talk the talk—they must walk the walk. Their actions should align with not only their values but yours as well. An ethically aligned relationship means you both are on the same page when it comes to integrity, kindness, and mutual respect. This ensures that your shared values create a strong bond.

Proof of Alliance

A great partner isn't just someone who enjoys the good times with you—they have your back in the tough moments too. Whether it's standing up for you or making sure your needs are met, they show you through their actions that you're a priority and that they're in your corner no matter what.

Energy.

Energy

Energy, in all its forms—physical, emotional, and spiritual—acts as the invisible force that fuels our daily lives. It's akin to the secret sauce in a recipe: without it, everything feels a little bland, or worse, utterly unpalatable. Let's break down how each type of energy can dramatically shape your day, and why the company you keep matters just as much as the energy you cultivate.

Imagine waking up after a fitful night's sleep, groggy and lethargic. That's physical fatigue—a heavy cloak that can wrap itself around you, making even the simplest tasks feel monumental. When your body is running on empty, your mind follows suit. You might find yourself struggling to concentrate, feeling irritable or, let's be honest, like a grumpy cat in a bath. Your productivity dips, and the world outside feels less vibrant, as if the colours have all been muted. The coffee you swore would be your saving grace becomes a fleeting fix rather than the sustaining fuel you need. The impact of physical fatigue extends beyond just feeling tired; it can cloud your judgement, making you more susceptible to emotional ups and downs, leaving you in a cycle of frustration.

Now let's talk about emotional fatigue—think of it as carrying a heavy backpack filled with stones that you just can't seem to shake off. When your emotional reserves are drained, you might find it challenging to engage with others or feel motivated to tackle your to-do list. The smallest inconveniences can trigger overwhelming feelings, and even the people you usually enjoy may suddenly seem insufferable. Emotionally fatigued, you may withdraw, cocooning yourself away from the world, which ironically can lead to feelings of loneliness that compound your fatigue. This emotional exhaustion acts like a fog, clouding your perception of the world and distorting the brightness of experiences that might otherwise be joyful.

Spiritual fatigue, while less talked about, can hit you like a ton of bricks. When your spirit feels depleted, your connection to purpose and meaning may falter. You might find yourself moving through the day as though you're on autopilot, devoid of the vibrant zest that makes life feel rich and fulfilling. The beauty in everyday moments can become obscured, and what once inspired you might now seem mundane. This disconnect can manifest as existential questions or a yearning for deeper connection, leaving you feeling adrift and longing for that sense of belonging.

But it's not just our own energy that affects us. The energy of those around us can act like a contagion, for better or worse. Positive, uplifting individuals can elevate your mood, making you feel like you're dancing on air, while those with negative or draining energy can leave you feeling heavy, much like a lead balloon. Imagine walking into a room filled with laughter and warmth—it's hard not to feel buoyed by that positive energy. Conversely, a room steeped in tension or negativity can feel stifling, as if someone has placed a weight on your chest. Surrounding yourself with positive stimuli—whether it's supportive friends, inspiring books or uplifting music—becomes essential for maintaining your energetic equilibrium and experiencing the world in a more vibrant light.

One of the most potent ways to revitalise all three types of energy is by immersing yourself in nature. The great outdoors acts as a powerful antidote to fatigue. Whether it's a stroll through a sun-dappled forest or simply sitting by a babbling brook, nature has a unique ability to ground us, restore balance and rejuvenate our spirits. The gentle rustling of leaves, the vibrant colours of blooming flowers and the soothing sounds of flowing water can breathe life back into your weary soul, offering an energetic reset. Nature invites us to pause, breathe deeply, and reconnect—not just with our surroundings, but with ourselves.

Energy is the lifeblood of our existence, intricately woven into the fabric of our daily experiences. By recognising the impact of physical, emotional, and spiritual fatigue on our lives, and by being mindful of the energy we allow to influence us, we can make choices that uplift and empower us. Surrounding ourselves with positive influences and nature's embrace isn't just a luxury; it's a necessity for thriving in a world that constantly demands our energy.

Take a moment today to check in with yourself and your surroundings—because your energy is not just your own; it's a vital part of the tapestry of life that connects us all. Remember, taking a break is what stops us from breaking.

Energy: Environment

Your environment isn't just a backdrop; it's the framework that shapes how you think, feel, and function. Imagine it as the architecture of your life—whether it's a sleek, modern design or a dilapidated fixer-upper is entirely up to you.

Picture this: you're attempting to concentrate in a room that's more landfill than living space—papers strewn everywhere, last week's coffee cup still lingering, and that lone sock you swore you'd find a match for. Hardly the setting for productivity? Now, contrast that with a space that's been thoughtfully arranged, where everything has its purpose, and suddenly, tackling even the most daunting tasks feels a bit more manageable.

How Your Environment Can Influence Your Mindset

1. **Mental Clarity:** A cluttered space leads to a cluttered mind, much like trying to navigate a maze with no exit. Streamlining your environment can help declutter your thoughts, allowing for clearer, more focused thinking.
2. **Mood Enhancement:** Your surroundings directly influence your mood. Filling your space with items that resonate with you—be it a well-chosen piece of art, a splash of greenery, or that perfect fragrance—can uplift your spirits and mitigate stress.
3. **Productivity Boost:** The right environment is like a custom-tailored suit—designed to fit your needs perfectly. Whether it's the ideal lighting, an ergonomically sound workspace, or an inspiring quote that actually speaks to you, these elements combine to create a space where you can thrive.

4. **Holistic Health:** A healthy environment transcends the physical realm to include emotional and social factors. Surround yourself with positive influences, both in your surroundings and your social circles, to enhance your overall well-being.

Crafting Your Ideal Environment

- **Declutter with Precision:** Regularly assess your space with the critical eye of a curator. A well-organised environment is the foundation upon which mental clarity and physical efficiency are built.

- **Personalise with Care:** Infuse your space with elements that speak to you on a deeper level. These are more than just decorations; they are reflections of your personality and contributors to your daily joy.

- **Design for Success:** Arrange your environment with purpose. Whether it's carving out a dedicated, distraction-free workspace or creating a serene corner for relaxation, your surroundings should be a deliberate extension of your goals and aspirations.

Your environment is not merely where you exist; it's the setting that influences how you perform. Whether it's the physical spaces you inhabit, the people you choose to be around, or the mental landscapes you cultivate, ensuring that your environment supports your goals is essential for thriving. Think of it as setting the stage for the life you want to lead—make sure the design is worthy of the performance.

Energy: Environment

Internal Environment

An internal safe space equips you to process emotions effectively, manage stress with grace, and build an anchor of resilience against life's inevitable storms. It's like having a mental toolkit that is always within reach and filled with the various strategies / tools that you require to navigate life's challenges. Through practices such as actively retraining your thoughts, identifying patterns of limiting beliefs and healing unresolved trauma, you can create a sanctuary within—a place where you find peace and clarity, no matter the chaos outside. It's like owning a secluded retreat in the wilderness where you can escape whenever the world becomes overwhelming.

The rewards of a supportive environment and a well-tended internal safe space are substantial. It boosts your confidence, allows you to navigate triggers with the grace of a ballet dancer, helps you maintain healthy boundaries, keeps you grounded, and instills a profound sense of security. With a strong internal refuge, you're better equipped to face life's ups and downs with resilience and poise. Surround yourself with reminders and positive influences, curate an uplifting mind and diligently nurture that inner sanctuary. When you become conscious of them, you can switch your thoughts from being the villains in your life, to your own personal team of superheroes, always ready to back you up and keep you steady. Remember, a supportive environment and a safe space aren't luxuries—they're essential to a life well-lived.

Energy: Environment

External Environment

Now, let's explore the great outdoors. Think of Mother Nature as the ultimate curator of peace and vitality—a rejuvenating force that offers the perfect antidote to the stressors of modern life. Spending time in nature is akin to hitting the reset button on your soul, and the benefits of this natural remedy are vast, making it well worth trading screen time for green time.

First, let's talk about fresh air. It's the ultimate tonic—pure, invigorating, and utterly free of side effects. When you breathe in the crisp air of the great outdoors, your lungs rejoice, your body feels revitalised, and your mind clears. It's nature's way of offering you a deep, calming breath and a gentle reminder to take things slow.

Secondly, sunshine. It is the equivalent to receiving a warm, comforting embrace from the universe, complete with a healthy dose of Vitamin D. Sunlight isn't just essential for strong bones and a resilient immune system; it also plays a crucial role in lifting your spirits. The sun's rays stimulate serotonin production, the hormone responsible for making you feel good, which is why a day spent in the sun leaves you feeling lighter and more content. Just don't forget the sunscreen—nobody wants to walk away from a lovely day outdoors looking like a boiled lobster.

Nature's beauty is unparalleled—think of it as the most exquisite art gallery, where every piece is a masterpiece crafted by time and the elements. From the vibrant hues of wildflowers to the soothing murmur of a babbling brook, nature has a way of easing your mind and sparking your creativity. Whether you're hiking through a dense forest, strolling along a sandy beach, or simply lying on the grass watching the clouds drift by, immersing yourself in nature offers a fresh perspective on life. It's your personal therapist who helps you find clarity without uttering a single word.

On the subject of therapy, did you know that nature is a powerful stress reliever? Studies have shown that spending time in natural settings can significantly lower stress levels, reduce anxiety, and even improve mental health. The next time you feel overwhelmed or a bit out of sorts, consider swapping your desk for a park bench and let the calming influence of nature work its magic. (I definitely have to remind myself to take my own advice on this one).

Let's not forget the physical benefits: Whether you're hiking, cycling, kayaking, or simply enjoying a leisurely walk, outdoor activities offer a far more enjoyable way to stay active than any gym routine. Plus, the bonus of breathtaking scenery and the occasional wildlife sighting (even if it's just a particularly bold squirrel) makes the experience all the more rewarding. Exercising in nature not only enhances your physical health but also gives you a mental boost, helping you feel more focused and energised.

Finally, spending time in nature fosters a connection to something greater than yourself. It serves as a gentle reminder that there's a vast, beautiful world out there, brimming with wonder and waiting to be explored. Whether you're watching a sunset, listening to the waves, or gazing at the stars, nature has a way of putting things into perspective and making your worries seem a little smaller.

Energy: Environment

Grab your hiking boots, pack a picnic, or simply bring along your sense of adventure, and head outdoors! Mother Nature is waiting, ready to share her bounty of benefits. Embrace the great outdoors, let the fresh air invigorate you, and bask in the natural beauty that surrounds you. After all, while there may be no Wi-Fi in the forest, you're sure to find a far more meaningful connection.

A little BONUS section for you on a new concept:

Neuroaesthetics

decoding our love for art and beauty.

Neuroaesthetics: Decoding Our Love for Art and Beauty

Picture this: you're strolling through an art gallery, latte in hand, Instagram-ready outfit on point. As you gaze at a stunning piece of modern art — maybe a giant abstract canvas that could easily be mistaken for a toddler's finger-painting project — your brain starts sending little love notes to itself. This is neuroaesthetics at work, the delightful intersection of neuroscience and aesthetics where art tangles with the inner workings of the brain.

Neuroaesthetics examines how our brains respond to beauty, transforming the fleeting thrill of a perfect sunset or a gorgeous bouquet from your lover into something tangible. It turns out that beauty isn't just in the eye of the beholder; it's a full-on brain spectacle! Our little noggin uses neural circuits to decode and process beauty, turning visual stimuli into an emotional experience that makes us feel all warm and fuzzy inside.

Let's break it down: certain areas of our brain light up in reaction to beauty — kind of how you might react when your crush just happens to like your latest Instagram post. The ventral striatum, a brain region associated with pleasure, goes full 'I-just-won-the-lottery' mode as it responds to aesthetically pleasing images. In simpler terms, your brain is flipping out, rewarding you with a little hit of dopamine everytime it sees something that it determines is pretty — the same feel-good chemical that's released when you eat your favourite dessert!

But why are we so captivated by beauty in all its various forms? Research suggests that our attraction to beauty, whether it's a stunning landscape or a perfectly arranged charcuterie board may relate to evolutionary advantages. Our ancestors after all were discerning when it came to selecting mates and habitats. A beautiful environment was a sign of resources and safety, making it the kind of place where you'd want to start a family (if not an Instagram influencer account).

In a world increasingly driven by screens, understanding neuroaesthetics can also help us navigate the endless barrage of visual information. It's not just about what looks good on social media; it's about how these aesthetics can impact our moods and mental states. A cosy coffee shop with warm lighting and tasteful art can provide the perfect backdrop for productivity, while stark neon signs in a bleak diner might be better suited for a dramatic movie scene than your next deep conversation.

While neuroaesthetics focuses heavily on the scientific side, we can't forget the artistry involved. Picture an artist armed with a palette bursting with colours, each stroke of their brush illuminating the chemistry happening inside our brains. When our eyes feast on a captivating painting or an evocative sculpture, our neurons are having their own private rave. The visual cortex kicks into high gear, translating shapes and colours into feelings that can make your heart race or your gut twist.

Studies have shown that engaging with art can reduce stress and anxiety, serving as an emotional release in the same way a good cry — or a binge-watch of your favourite guilty pleasures — might do.
What's even more fascinating is how this connection to art can foster empathy. Have you ever been moved by a photograph that captured raw human emotion? That feeling might prompt you to act more compassionately in daily life, proving that our brains are wired not just to appreciate beauty, but to connect it to our social existence. Art shows us perspectives, allows us to walk in another's shoes (or Gucci slides, if you prefer) and enhances our capacity for understanding.

Neuroaesthetics: Decoding Our Love for Art and Beauty

As you delve into your daily life, whether strolling through an art exhibit, scrolling through your Pinterest inspiration board, or even curating your social media aesthetics, remember that neuroaesthetics is all about the delightful interplay between beauty, emotion, and the brain. It invites you to appreciate not just how art looks, but how it makes you feel — a reminder that beauty is not merely superficial; it's deeply interwoven into our emotional fabric. Whether it is a waterfall, a beach, a night at the ballet, a night with your beautiful lover, an art gallery or simply a cute little cafe that kind of feels like home, you can capitalise on this wonderful neural integration of yours by actively taking yourself to places that hold that little bit of awe.

The next time you catch your breath at an art piece or find yourself enchanted by a beautifully styled flat lay, know that your brain is celebrating alongside you! After all, in the grand gallery of life, we're all just trying to curate our own unique collections of joy, beauty, and connection. So, sip that latte, absorb those visuals, and let your neurons dance to their own aesthetic beat!

Energy: Exercise

A quick yet important note on movement: As you dive into processing trauma and regulating your nervous system, don't be surprised if your relationship with movement takes a sharp left turn. For years, I was all about the "no pain, no gain" life—pushing my body to its limits with high-intensity workouts and convincing myself it was therapy. Spoiler: it wasn't. Once I started doing the actual work of healing, my body gave me a clear message: "Enough of that nonsense." Suddenly, I wasn't craving the gym grind. Yoga became my best friend, slow walks replaced frantic cardio, and deep, meditative breathing felt more satisfying than planking my way to oblivion. Even the idea of skipping a second workout in favour of rest didn't send me into a spiral—it was revolutionary. And you know what? My whole vibe shifted. Calm. Present. Actually enjoying the stillness.

Now, your journey might look completely different. Maybe you're currently in team "sloth mode," and as you heal, you'll find yourself itching to move. Or maybe you're somewhere in between. Whatever your body asks for, listen. Honour its cues like the queen you are. Your body isn't out to sabotage you—it's handing you the map to what it really needs. And trust me, when you start following it, the shifts are undeniable. Healing isn't about forcing yourself into someone else's routine; it's about owning your journey and finding the kind of movement that makes you feel alive.

Energy: Exercise

Exercise... or as I like to call it, the magical art of sweating out toxins, toxic behaviour, toxic energy, and most importantly, toxic attachments.

First, let's talk about the sweat strategy. For my hormonal imbalance babes, firstly, I am sending you so much love because this sh*t is no joke! Secondly, let's face it, sometimes exercise and movement are just not our BFFs—especially when the Endo or Adeno belly hits and makes you feel like a human balloon. Even for fitness enthusiasts, there are days when the body screams for 'active' rest. Sweat is a way to get that coveted endorphin hit without needing to go full-on workout mode. High temperatures from a sauna or good ol' sunshine trigger the body to release endorphins, those delightful chemicals that help decrease pain and discomfort from symptom flare-ups. On days when you can't bend into a downward dog or even muster the energy to walk, a sauna or some sunshine can be your go-to.

When you're feeling like a bloated balloon my love, focus on active rest. It's all about gentle movements and activities that soothe your body:

- **Acupuncture:** Needles may sound scary, but they can be a game-changer for pain relief and relaxation.

- **Massage:** Treat yourself to a massage to melt away tension and improve circulation.

- **Sauna:** Let the heat work its magic by detoxifying and reducing inflammation.

- **Sunshine:** Bask in the sun's warm embrace to boost your mood and soak up some vitamin D.

Energy: Exercise

- **Mobility-Focused Movement:** Gentle stretches and mobility exercises keep muscles warm and engaged without overexerting yourself.

- **Laying in bed with a heat pack and crying if you need to.** I totally understand how debilitating the pain can be when it really hits, I just wish that I could give you the biggest hug and take all of that pain away. I might not be able to magically remove that pain for you right now, but together, with the right lifestyle changes, nutrition, deep healing and consistency, we can definitely get it to a minimum. I believe in you, and me... I believe in us!

Anti-Inflammatory Activities: These activities help calm your nervous system and reduce inflammation, making them perfect for when you need to unwind:

- **Yin Yoga:** Slow, deep stretches that target the connective tissues and promote relaxation.

- **Qigong:** This ancient Chinese practice combines gentle movement, meditation, and breathing exercises to balance your energy.

- **Yoga:** Whether it's a gentle flow or restorative practice, yoga can help you connect with your body and mind.

- **Walking Outdoors:** A simple walk in nature can do wonders for your mood and overall well-being.

Energy: Exercise

Movement isn't just about physical benefits; it's also a powerful way to release emotions:

- **Shaking:** Let loose and shake off the stress and tension.
- **Dancing:** Put on your favourite tunes and dance like nobody's watching.
- **Tapping:** Use EFT (Emotional Freedom Techniques) to tap on acupressure points and release emotional blocks.
- **Walk and Talk:** Sometimes, a chat with a non-biased friend can help you step out of your own tunnel vision and see the bigger picture.

Side note: Meditation and green juice are great for supporting your body, but let's not kid ourselves—they won't single-handedly prevent burnout. Think of them as premium fuel for your car: they'll optimise performance and help you feel fantastic, but if you keep driving without stopping to refuel, it doesn't matter how premium the petrol is—you'll still end up stranded on the side of the road when the tank runs dry. Rest and recovery aren't optional extras; they're non-negotiables.

Remember, it's not about forcing yourself to hit the gym every day. It's about finding what feels good for your body and aligning with each phase of your cycle. Whether it's sweating it out in a sauna, moving gently with yoga, or shaking off stress with a dance party, listen to your body and give it the love and care it deserves.

Implementing Space.

Implementing Space

The word 'growth' has become the equivalent of your favourite pair of jeans—overused, but let's be honest, not something you're ready to toss just yet. It's always there when you need it, holding everything together while still giving you room to breathe.

We talk about growth like it's this grand, glittery ideal, but what does it really mean? Think of it less as a vague, feel-good mantra and more as a personal Marie Kondo for your life. Instead of deciding if that old sweater "sparks joy," you're taking a hard look at your habits and routines—because let's face it, some of them have seriously outstayed their welcome.

So, where does your time go? No, really—where? If your screen time report is trying to send you an intervention or you're watching a series that should've ended two seasons ago, we have a problem. Step one in this growth glow-up is recognising where your precious minutes are slipping away, and taking them back one scroll at a time.

Now that you've located the time leaks, let's talk about what actually matters to you. Learning a new skill? Getting your fitness on? Quality time with friends? Finally launching that side hustle? Write it all down, prioritise, and prepare to make some room. Because here's the truth: if you want change, you have to make space for it.

Which brings us to the inevitable: scheduling. Yes, it may sound like the least exciting thing since watching your hair air-dry, but it's key. Block out specific time for the activities that will get you closer to who you want to become, because if you don't schedule it, it won't happen. Start small—just 10 minutes a day—then work your way up. Maybe take a weekend to focus on yourself, or go big with a week off to dive into something new. The goal is to create more time for the future you and less time for the current you that's stuck in the same loop. After all, repeating the same routine and expecting change? Well, that's the definition of insanity.

Once that sacred growth time is in your calendar, guard it as if it's your most coveted invite. Tell your friends you're off the grid, turn on aeroplane mode, and eliminate distractions. This is your time for growth—treat it as a non-negotiable meeting with your future self. Remember, you don't have to become a "productivity queen", this is not about jamming your calender, it is about removing anything that does not reciprocate the energy that you put into it. This exercise should free up your time to be used by what makes your life fulfilling.

I highly encourage using this exercise to block out time to do absolutely nothing, rest, simply be and exist. Start with small, manageable chunks—maybe a quick workout or 15 minutes of sitting and breathing each morning. The important thing is consistency, not perfection. Rome wasn't built in a day, and neither are life-changing habits.

Of course, life has a funny way of laughing at your plans. You'll need to adjust, flex, and pivot—just make sure you return to your routine as soon as possible. Balance is key, not burnout.

Implementing Space

At the end of the week, give yourself a quick debrief. What worked? What didn't? Refine and adjust. Growth is less about grand gestures and more about those small, consistent tweaks that push you forward. When you hit those milestones? Celebrate—because who doesn't deserve a little confetti now and then?

Here's the real takeaway: creating space for growth isn't about stuffing more into your already packed schedule. It's about making smart, intentional choices that carve out room for what actually matters. Audit your time, set your priorities, and create space for the life you want. Because at the end of the day, you don't rise to the level of your goals—you fall to the level of your habits. Five-year plans are great, but without the daily commitment to back them up, they're just wishful thinking. Make space for the person you want to be, and watch how quickly that change becomes your new reality.

Journal Prompts.

Journal Prompts

CONGRATULATIONS!

You did it! Congratulations on completing this journey. As a little gift to celebrate, I've included an extra section in this book filled with journal prompts designed to help you process beliefs and dive into neural and emotional rewiring. These prompts are here for you to explore at your own pace, using the notes pages that follow.

Take as much time and space as you need with each prompt—there's no rush and no rules. Rather than pre-setting them out, I wanted to give you the freedom to use them however feels right for you. This is your space to reflect, rewire, and grow.

Neural Rewiring Journal Prompts:

Pros vs. Cons

Sometimes, the simplest tools can unlock the biggest breakthroughs. Understanding the benefits and drawbacks of your habits is a pivotal first step in implementing change. Grab a pen, make two columns, and list the pros and cons of the habit you want to break. This isn't just about seeing what you're losing—it's about discovering what you stand to gain.

I know, it might sound too simple, even obvious. That's exactly what I thought when my mentor suggested this exercise as I wrestled with an eating adaptation (formerly known as a disorder) that had gripped me for nine years. My initial response? An eye roll so dramatic it probably counted as cardio. "There are no pros," I snapped. "I hate it, I want to get rid of it, it ruins my life." Calmly, he replied: "If there were no pros, you wouldn't still be doing it."

That response stopped me in my tracks. Taking the time to list the pros forced me to confront the real reasons I was holding on. Slowly, I started to see that each so-called "pro" of this maladaptive behaviour could be achieved in healthier, more nourishing ways. With that clarity, I was able to let go of the habit, not by force, but by understanding and replacing it with something that truly served me. This isn't just a hack—it's a revelation. Try it, and you might be surprised by what you uncover.

Trigger Journal

Every time you feel the pull of a habit you're trying to break, pause and take inventory of the moment. What's happening around you? Who are you with? What's running through your mind? Who—or what—is taking up your mental space? What's your current environment, or what's about to change? These moments hold invaluable clues. By observing them, you'll start to see patterns emerge, revealing the triggers behind your behaviour.

For me, this process was a game-changer in understanding my eating disorder. I had always assumed that growing up in a ballet studio was the root cause of my disordered eating. Ballet, with its intense focus on perfection, seemed like the obvious villain. As I began tracking my triggers, a different picture emerged. I noticed I could walk in and out of a dance studio without issue. The real problems arose when a certain person in my life was about to visit. Suddenly, the critical thoughts flooded in, and anxiety fuelled the behaviour. It wasn't ballet—it was this person.

Avoidance might have seemed like the easy solution, but I knew that cutting them out wouldn't truly resolve the issue. Instead, I faced it head-on. I had a deeply uncomfortable, brutally honest conversation about how their presence and words were affecting me. It wasn't easy, and it didn't fix things overnight, but over time, through processing and courage, that trigger lost its power.

The lesson? Sometimes, it's not about avoiding the trigger; it's about understanding and addressing it. Only then can you truly begin to break free.

Old Thought | New Thought

Old Thought:
Ugh, I have to...

New Thought:
I'm so grateful that I get to...

Sometimes replacing an old thought is as simple as flipping a switch. Other times, it's more like rewiring an entire circuit. When those stubborn, deep-rooted beliefs arise, take a moment to get curious:

What is this thought trying to achieve?
What do I need to learn in order to let it go?
What part of me is holding on to this?
How can I show this part of myself more love and compassion?
Where did this thought or belief originate?
Does it still serve me?
I ask myself, how can I help you?

If the thought isn't anchored in a highly charged emotional trigger and you feel safe exploring, revisit the memory where it first took root. With the wisdom and perspective you have now, rewrite the story. Shift the narrative into something that empowers you, rather than limits you.

If this feels overwhelming or uncertain, that's ok. Working with a trauma-informed practitioner can provide the safety and guidance needed to navigate and rewrite these stories effectively, ensuring the process supports your growth rather than re-traumatising.

Daily Journal
Take time each day to get acquainted with your own mind. Journaling allows you to explore hidden thoughts, uncover subconscious beliefs, and identify patterns that might otherwise go unnoticed. Over time, it becomes a powerful tool to chart your growth and gain clarity. Think of it as a safe, non-judgemental space to sift through the noise and truly understand yourself on a deeper level.

Swap, Don't Stop | Micro Changes
Habits are stubborn little neural pathways, but you don't have to bulldoze them to make a change. Instead of cutting them off cold turkey, ease the transition by swapping the habit for something similar—but healthier or more productive.

Take caffeine, for example. When I need a break, I don't quit the ritual of a morning drink—I just swap coffee for ginger tea. If that doesn't cut it, I meet myself halfway with a matcha latte, which offers a gentler caffeine kick. It turns out, it's usually not the coffee itself that I crave but the comfort of a warm drink to start my day. Even when working in cafes, I didn't stop showing up—I just swapped my coffee order for something non-caffeinated. The environment and routine stayed the same.

The same goes for other habits. When I gave up alcohol for a year, I didn't sit at home sulking. I swapped my go-to drink for a mocktail or sparkling water in a fancy glass. It wasn't the alcohol I missed; it was the ritual—the sense of indulgence in a social setting.

Ask yourself: What's one small tweak you can make to keep the ritual alive while breaking the habit? It's these micro changes that pave the way for lasting transformation.

Fact-Check Your Thoughts

Here's where we put your thoughts on trial: Are they based on fear, or are they grounded in fact? Start by writing down the thought that's nagging at you. What's driving it? What are you afraid of? Now, imagine standing in a courtroom—would this thought hold up under cross-examination? Would it pass the test of truth?

This is where the Old Thought | New Thought technique comes in. Take the fear-based thought and re-frame it using new, empowering truths. For instance:
Old Thought: "I always mess things up."
New Thought: "I've learned from past mistakes and grown because of them."

Fear thrives on assumptions, while facts give you clarity. By fact-checking your thoughts and rewriting the script, you can shift from limiting beliefs to ones that serve your growth. It's not about silencing the inner critic—it's about giving it better material to work with.

A Personal Note.

A Personal Note

As I write these final words, I'm not here to tie it all up with a neat little bow. Healing isn't neat, and it's never linear. What I hope this book has given you isn't answers but a mirror—a way to see yourself more clearly, with honesty and compassion. I hope it's loosened the grip of self-blame just enough for you to catch your breath and see your body not as the enemy, but as something trying—however messily—to protect you.

Writing this book for you, has been its own reckoning for me. I've spent so much of my life feeling betrayed by my body, at war with its unpredictability, its pain, its refusal to just be normal. As I started to sit with this new information, I began to realise that my body wasn't sabotaging me—it was screaming for help. Every imbalance, every crash, every moment that I felt like I was falling apart was my body's way of waving a flag, begging me to listen. It wasn't trying to hurt me, it was trying to save me.

Looking back at my darkest moments in life, I can see now how deeply my hormones and nervous system shaped this experience—my thoughts, my moods, my ability to even function. When those systems were out of sync, life itself felt unmanageable. Was it the chaos of my life that threw everything off balance, or was it the imbalance that made life feel so chaotic? Honestly, I don't know. What I do know is that the answer didn't come from trying to "fix" myself but from finally sitting down and paying attention.

Here's the truth: this work is hard. It's not glamorous, and it doesn't come with quick fixes, Instagrammable milestones or even Christmas bonuses (I am typing this in December). Some days, it will feel like nothing's changing. Other days, it will feel like everything's cracking open. The one thing I can promise you is that it's worth it. Learning to care for yourself—not in the performative, self-care Sundays way, but in the raw, gritty, show-up-for-yourself-when-it's-hard way—is the most profound shift you'll ever make.

Caring for your mind and body isn't a luxury, a chore, or something to squeeze into the cracks of a busy life—it's the cornerstone of everything else. It's not about punishing routines or chasing perfection; it's about balance, it's about finding the grace to breathe through the messy, human moments. It's about turning your inner voice from a relentless judge into a kind companion, because no matter where life takes you, that voice will always be there. Let it be one that lifts you, one you'd actually want to listen to. You deserve that.

I'm not here to tell you that you're going to wake up one day and everything will be fine. That's not real, and we both know it. What I am here to say is that every small choice to listen to yourself, every moment you stop to ask what you need, every time you soften instead of judge—that's where the change happens. Not overnight, but over time.

Thank you for trusting me enough to make it to this point. If nothing else, I hope this book has reminded you that you're not alone in this. That your messiness, your struggle, your humanity—it's all part of it. And it's enough. You are enough.

With all my love,
NJT. x

Index:

Now that you have trusted the process, here is an actual index for your own reference:

This book has been proofed and backed by Dr. Ces Franks

Dr. Ces Franks is a distinguished expert in integrative medicine with nearly six decades of experience across multiple disciplines. Beginning his career as a psychologist specializing in trauma, he developed a deep understanding of the mind's role in healing and resilience. After a decade in psychology, Dr. Franks expanded his expertise to include chiropractic care, naturopathy, osteopathy, iridology, and biomechanics. This rare and comprehensive skill set positions him uniquely as a leader in healthcare.

In 1975, Dr. Franks established Vital Life Clinics, a pioneering health center dedicated to delivering whole-person care. Through Vital Life Clinics, Dr. Franks has served thousands of patients, applying evidence-based practices and a unique blend of traditional and natural therapies to address both acute and chronic conditions. Known for his profound expertise and commitment to the science of healing, Dr. Franks has built a reputation for restoring health and vitality from the inside out, setting a gold standard in integrative wellness.

References:

Australian Bureau of Statistics (2023). Recorded Crime - Victims. [online] www.abs.gov.au. Available at: https://www.abs.gov.au/statistics/people/crime-and-justice/recorded-crime-victims/latest-release.

Bartlett, S. (2023). The Diary of a CEO. Penguin.

Bollu, P.C. and Kaur, H. (2019). Sleep Medicine: Insomnia and Sleep. Missouri Medicine, [online] 116(1), p.68. Available at: https://pmc.ncbi.nlm.nih.gov/articles/PMC6390785/ [Accessed 17 Oct. 2024].

Glazer, N. (2008). Purposeful Youth. [online] Education Next. Available at: https://www.educationnext.org/purposeful-youth/ [Accessed 13 Oct. 2024].

Inc, S. (n.d.). Top 12 Health and Wellness Benefits of Sauna. [online] www.finnleo.com. Available at: https://www.finnleo.com/pages/health-and-wellness#:~:text=Under%20the%20high%2Dheat%20provided.

Johnson, R. (2020). The Impact of Unresolved Trauma on Relationships. [online] A New Outlook Recovery Services. Available at: https://coloradorecoveryservices.org/the-impact-of-unresolved-trauma-on-relationships/.

Judith Lewis Herman (1992). Trauma and recovery : the aftermath of violence--from domestic abuse to political terror. New York: Basic Books.

Mayo Clinic (2016). Insomnia treatment: Cognitive behavioral therapy instead of sleeping pills. [online] Mayo Clinic. Available at: https://www.mayoclinic.org/diseases-conditions/insomnia/in-depth/insomnia-treatment/art-20046677.

Michaud, M. (2019). Not All Sleep is Equal When It Comes to Cleaning the Brain. [online] URMC Newsroom. Available at: https://www.urmc.rochester.edu/news/story/not-all-sleep-is-equal-when-it-comes-to-cleaning-the-brain.

Mindfulness Matters (2017). Mindfulness Matters. [online] NIH News in Health. Available at: https://newsinhealth.nih.gov/2012/01/mindfulness-matters.

Oxford Languages (2024). Oxford Languages. [online] Oxford Languages. Available at: https://languages.oup.com/google-dictionary-en/.

Pesetsky, J. (2020). Healthy Relationships in Practice. [online] The Gottman Institute. Available at: https://www.gottman.com/blog/healthy-relationships-in-practice/.

Psychology Today. (2023). 3 Common Pitfalls of Unresolved Trauma in Relationships. [online] Available at: https://www.psychologytoday.com/au/blog/understanding-ptsd/202310/3-common-pitfalls-of-unresolved-trauma-in-relationships#:~:text=Some%20of%20the%20more%20common [Accessed 4 Aug. 2024].

Puderbaugh, M. and Emmady, P.D. (2023). Neuroplasticity. [online] National Library of Medicine. Available at: https://www.ncbi.nlm.nih.gov/books/NBK557811/.

Rosenberg, M.B. (2003). Nonviolent communication : a language of compassion. Del Mar, Ca: Puddledancer Press.

Scottsdale Community College (2019). Why Having a Sense of Purpose is Important | Scottsdale Community College. [online] www.scottsdalecc.edu. Available at: https://www.scottsdalecc.edu/news/2019/why-having-sense-purpose-important.

Shetty, M. (2023). How Social Connection Supports Longevity | Social Engagement. [online] Lifestyle Medicine. Available at: https://longevity.stanford.edu/lifestyle/2023/12/18/how-social-connection-supports-longevity/.

Van Der Kolk, B. (2014). The body keeps the score: Brain, mind, and body in the healing of trauma. New York, New York: Penguin Books.

Wein, H. (2021). Good sleep for good health. [online] NIH News in Health. Available at: https://newsinhealth.nih.gov/2021/04/good-sleep-good-health.

Notes:

Notes:

Notes:

Notes:

Notes:

Notes:

Notes:

Notes:

Notes:

Notes:

Notes:

Notes:

Notes:

Made in the USA
Monee, IL
10 November 2026

449de253-ca0a-44c6-9f2f-c2d9028e28a4R01